Grief Diaries

SURVIVING LOSS OF AN INFANT

True heartfelt stories about surviving the aftermath of losing an infant

LYNDA CHELDELIN FELL
with
LINDA BATEMAN GOMEZ
MARY LEE CLAFLIN

FOREWORD BY
LINDA BATEMAN GOMEZ
Parent Day Council National Parent of the Year

Grief Diaries
Surviving Loss of an Infant – 1ST ed.
True heartfelt stories about surviving the aftermath of losing an infant.
Lynda Cheldelin Fell/Linda Bateman-Gomez/Mary Lee Claflin
Grief Diaries www.GriefDiaries.com

Cover Design by AlyBlue Media, LLC
Interior Design by AlyBlue Media LLC
Published by AlyBlue Media, LLC

ISBN: 978-1-944328-04-7
Library of Congress Control Number: 2015916915
AlyBlue Media, LLC
Ferndale, WA 98248
www.AlyBlueMedia.com

This book is designed to provide informative narrations to readers. It is sold with the understanding that the writers, authors or publisher is not engaged to render any type of psychological, legal, or any other kind of professional advice. The content is the sole expression and opinion of the authors and writers. No warranties or guarantees are expressed or implied by the choice to include any of the content in this book. Neither the publisher nor the author or writers shall be liable for any physical, psychological, emotional, financial, or commercial damages including but not limited to special, incidental, consequential or other damages. Our views and rights are the same: You are responsible for your own choices, actions and results.

PRINTED IN THE UNITED STATES OF AMERICA

TESTIMONIALS

"CRITICALLY IMPORTANT . . . *I want to say to Lynda that what you are doing is so critically important.*"
–DR. BERNICE A. KING, Daughter of Dr. Martin Luther King

"INSPIRATIONAL . . . *Grief Diaries: Loss by Impaired Driving is the result of heartfelt testimonials from a dedicated and loving group of people. By sharing their stories, the reader will learn the true devastation that impaired driving causes, and perhaps find inspiration and a renewed sense of comfort as they move through their own journey.*" -CANDACE LIGHTNER, Founder of Mothers Against Drunk Driving

"DEEPLY INTIMATE . . . Grief Diaries *is a deeply intimate, authentic collection of narratives that speak to the powerful, often ambiguous, and wide spectrum of emotions that arise from loss. I so appreciate the vulnerability and truth embedded in these stories, which honor and bear witness to the many forms of bereavement that arise in the aftermath of death.*" -DR. ERICA GOLDBLATT HYATT, Chair of Psychology, Bryn Athyn College

"MOVING . . . *We learn from stories throughout life. In Grief Diaries, the stories are not only moving but often provide a rich background for any mourner to find a gem of insight that can be used in coping with loss. Reread each story with pen in hand and you will find many that are just right for you.*" -DR. LOUIS LAGRAND, Author of Healing Grief, Finding Peace

"VITAL . . . *Grief Diaries: Surviving Loss of a Pregnancy gives voice to the thousands of women who face this painful journey every day. Often alone in their time of need, these stories will play a vital role in surrounding each reader with warmth and comfort as they seek understanding and healing in the aftermath of their own loss.*" -JENNIFER CLARKE, obstetrical R.N., Perinatal Bereavement Committee at AMITA Health Adventist Medical Center, founder of Baby Jasmine's Angel Nursery and advocate of CuddleCots

"A FORCE . . . *The writers of this project, the Grief Diaries anthology series, are a force to be reckoned with. I'm betting we will be agents of great change.*" -MARY LEE ROBINSON, Author and Founder of Set an Extra Plate initiative

"HEALING . . . *Grief Diaries: Surviving Loss of a Pregnancy gives voice to a grief so private, most women bear it alone. These diaries of pregnancy loss can heal hearts and begin to build community and acceptance to speak the unspeakable, to acknowledge each pregnancy loss and the child that would have been. Share this book with your sisters, mothers, grandmothers and friends who have faced the grief of pregnancy loss. Pour a cup of tea together and know that you are no longer alone.*" -DIANNA VAGIANOS ARMENTROUT, Poetry Therapist & Author of *Walking the Labyrinth of My Heart*: *A Journey of Pregnancy, Grief and Infant Death*

"INCREDIBLE . . . *Thank you so much for doing this project, it's absolutely incredible!*"-JULIE MJELVE, Founder, Grieving Together

"STUNNING . . . *Grief Diaries treats the reader to a rare combination of candor and fragility through the eyes of the bereaved. Delving into the deepest recesses of the heartbroken, the reader easily identifies with the diverse collection of stories and richly colored threads of profound love that create a stunning read full of comfort and hope.*" -DR. GLORIA HORSLEY, President, Open to Hope Foundation

"WONDERFUL . . . *Grief Diaries is a wonderful computation of stories written by the best of experts, the bereaved themselves. Thank you for building awareness about a topic so near and dear to my heart.*"
-DR. HEIDI HORSLEY, Adjunct Professor, School of Social Work, Columbia University, Author, Co-Founder of Open to Hope Organization

"HOPE AND HEALING . . . *You are a pioneer in this field and you are breaking the trail for others to find hope and healing.*"
-KRISTI SMITH, Bestselling Author & International Speaker

"GLOBAL . . . *One of The Five Facets of Healing mantras is together we can heal a world of hurt. This anthology series is testimony to the power we have as global neighbors to do just that.*"
-ANNAH ELIZABETH, Founder of The Five Facets of Healing

SURVIVING LOSS OF AN INFANT

DEDICATION

To our beloved children:
Moments are fleeting,
memories are permanent,
love is forever.

Gavin Michael
Brimley Shyanne Barks
Chad Ernest Gomez
Taylor Reanne Kaup
Lane Edward Lawson
Elijah Luna
William Oscar Mead
Diego Ramon Romero
Dominique "Deedee" Faith St. George
Anthony James Williams

CONTENTS

FOREWORD

The loss of a child is by far one of the most incomprehensible tragedies anyone can go through. It can challenge everything you believe in and leave even the strongest, weak. If you fall into this painful category, my heart breaks for you and your family, as I have been there.

When I lost my son in 1986, I felt as though my world had ended. Despite having an incredible support system, to this day, it remains one of the most difficult times of my life.

Everyone's grieving process is different and for each there will be varied, and sometimes unexpected, challenges along the path of healing including well intended sympathizers that perhaps say the wrong thing, marital challenges, anniversaries of birthdays and death, and many others. The pages that follow are a shared collection of stories and experiences from those who have been in your very position. Each writer has opened their heart in service to this book, to help you find ways to navigate through the grief and ease some of the challenges you face during this time.

Finally, the one overarching message that we hope you take away from this book is a message of hope. As difficult as life may be now, the pain does ease and things do get better. There is hope for happiness after your loss, and this book represents an entire community that stands with you in your grief, knows your strengths, and can help you through.

Many blessings,
Linda Bateman Gomez xoxo

PREFACE

One night in 2007, I had one of *those* dreams, the vivid kind you can't shake. In the dream, I was the front passenger in a car and my daughter Aly was sitting behind the driver. Suddenly, the car missed a curve in the road and sailed into a lake. The driver and I escaped the sinking car, but Aly did not. Desperately flailing through the deep murky water to find my daughter, I failed. She was gone. Aly was gone. The only evidence left behind was an open book floating where my beloved daughter disappeared.

Two years later that nightmare became reality when my daughter died as a back seat passenger in a car accident on August 5, 2009. She was just fifteen years old.

I now understand that the dream two years before Aly's death was a glimpse into a divine plan that would eventually touch many lives. The book left floating on the water was actually a peek at my future. But the devastation I felt in my heart would blind me to the meaning of that dream for a long time to come.

In the aftermath of losing Aly, I eventually discovered that helping others was a powerful way to heal my own heart. There is nothing more beautiful than one extending compassion and comfort to another in need. The Grief Diaries series was born and built on this belief. By writing books narrating our journeys through hardship and losses, our written words become a portable support group for others. When we swap stories, we feel less alone. It is comforting to know someone else understands the shoes we walk in, and the challenges we face along the way.

Which brings us to this book, *Grief Diaries: Surviving Loss of an Infant.* The devastation left in the aftermath of losing a baby, no matter how small, can steal your breath, and leave you with more questions than answers. Further, you might encounter people who don't understand your emotions or, worse, lack compassion for your journey. This is where the *Grief Diaries* series can help.

Helen Keller once said, "Walking with a friend in the dark is better than walking alone in the light." This is especially true in the aftermath of loss. If you have lost an infant, the following true stories are written by courageous women who know exactly how you feel, for they've been in your shoes and have walked the same path. Perhaps the shoes are a different size or style, but may you find comfort in these stories and the understanding that you aren't truly alone on the journey. For we walk ahead, behind, and right beside you.

Wishing you healing, and hope from the Grief Diaries village.

Warm regards,

Lynda Cheldelin Fell

Creator, Grief Diaries

BY LYNDA CHELDELIN FELL

THE WAILING TENT

Dear grieving mother,

Welcome to the sisterhood of the wailing tent. Although with profound condolences, I know this greeting will soon be forgotten, for your heart and soul have sustained a terrible blow. The shock known as "the fog" will accompany you for some time, greatly impacting your memory. So I offer you this written welcome to refer to when your recollection falters.

The wailing tent is an honored place where only mothers with a broken spirit can enter. Admittance is gained not with an ID card bearing your name, but with the profound sorrow freshly etched on your heart. Membership is free, for you have already paid the unfathomable price. The directions to the wailing tent are secret, available only to mothers who speak our language of everlasting grief. No rules are posted, no hours are noted. There is no hierarchy, no governing body. Your membership has no expiration date; it is lifelong.

The refuge offered within its walls does not judge members based on age, religious belief, or social status. You can hang your mask outside and, if you can't make it past the door, we will surround you with love right where you lay.

The wailing tent is a shelter where mothers shed anguished tears among their comforting sisters. It is a haven where all forms of wailing are honored, understood, and accepted. In the beginning, you will be very afraid, and will hate the wailing tent and everything it stands for. You will flail, thrash about, and spew vile words in protest. You will fight to be free of the walls, wishing desperately to offer a plea bargain for a different tent, learn a different language. Those emotions will last for some time.

Your family and friends cannot accompany you here. The needs of the wailing tent are invisible to them and, though they will frantically try, they simply cannot comprehend the language nor fathom the disembodied, guttural howls heard within.

In the beginning, your stays here will seem endless. Over time, the need for your visits will change and eventually you will observe some mothers talking, even smiling, rather than wailing. Those are the mothers who have learned to balance profound anguish with moments of peace, though they still need to seek refuge among us from time to time. Do not judge those mothers as callused or strong, for they have endured profound heartache to attain the peace they have found. Their visits here are greatly valued, for their hard- earned wisdom offers hope that we too will learn to balance the sadness in our hearts.

Finally, you need not flash your ID card or introduce yourself each time you visit, for we know who you are. You are one of us, a lifelong sister of the wailing tent.

Welcome, my wailing sister.

Fondly,
The Sisterhood of the Wailing Tent

CHAPTER ONE

THE BEGINNING

Tears have a wisdom all their own. They come when a person has relaxed enough to let go to work through his sorrow. They are the natural bleeding of an emotional wound, carrying the poison out of the system. Here lies the road to recovery.
-F. ALEXANDER MAGOUN

Grief and sorrow is as unique to each individual as his or her fingerprint. In order to fully appreciate one's perspective, it is helpful to understand one's journey. In this chapter each writer shares that moment when they lost their precious baby to help you understand when life as they knew it ended, and a new one began.

*

DIANNA VAGIANOS ARMENTROUT
Dianna lost her newborn baby
Mary Rose in 2014 to trisomy 18

I have been pregnant four times. I have one living child. My second pregnancy, with my daughter, Mary Rose, was my first pregnancy loss. At the routine mid-pregnancy ultrasound, we found out that she had a fatal chromosomal disorder. I carried her to term not knowing if she would be born still or living. She was born on August 8, 2014, and died an hour after birth. About a year after her birth and death I had two early miscarriages, one in July and one in October. I assumed because I had carried one healthy child and one fatally ill child to term that I would do so again. The miscarriage in July was not too upsetting because I didn't feel very pregnant. My sense of smell wasn't like it was in my first two pregnancies. My breasts did not ache, and I thought that something wasn't right. I had some pregnancy symptoms, but did not feel the acceleration of hormones I had felt during my first two pregnancies. Even an early miscarriage is painful. I had afterpains and birthed a membrane. The next pregnancy in October was the first planned conception for me and for my husband. The hormones kicked in and I felt very sick. When I miscarried this second pregnancy at about the same time period, five weeks of pregnancy, I was devastated.

As my husband and I are older parents, this is particularly difficult to process. We have one living son but would like for him to have a sibling. We didn't choose our path, although Mary Rose is a gift that we treasure. I wish that I had another two years to mourn her and the miscarriages, to gather my courage to consider another pregnancy, but we don't have that kind of time. Since I have a lot of trauma around pregnancy and newborns, the best that I can do is to leave the door open without making any attempts at another pregnancy. "I want whatever God wants" Byron Katie says in her book *Loving What Is*. I want whatever God wants; I pray.

My pregnancy with Mary Rose was so stressful and difficult. I was in shock and was grief-stricken. My body became full of pain. I had sciatica, hip and back pain. I planned her funeral while I was pregnant. Though my body wanted to nest and prepare a nursery, we bought a plot and a casket. I met with a neonatologist and a pediatric cardiologist. I had hospice involved. When the nurse manager tried to destroy my plan to labor at home, my back went out, so I could only limp around in extreme pain. My body felt the way my soul was feeling. I was stuck, unable to move forward. I knew that once I labored, my baby would die. Not all babies with trisomy 18 die; there are two hundred in this country over one year of age. But I knew Mary Rose was not going to stay with us.

It took me a long time to figure out how to birth her at home. We needed a signed Do Not Resuscitate Order, a licensed midwife, and a pediatrician who was willing to make a house call to diagnose Mary Rose at birth. I wanted a quiet birth for the brief time that we would have with her, and her trisomy 18 posed no additional risk to me. I wanted my toddler to meet his sister. I wanted to prepare my daughter's body for her funeral without her body going through the morgue. This took incredible advocacy and stubborn love. We did it.

Mary Rose was born in a pool at home under a painting entitled "Healing Companion," that my friend Sindy Strosahl made of my daughter and me when I was pregnant. In the painting, my daughter is an angel standing behind me tenderly holding her serious, pregnant mother.

I prepared Mary Rose's body and we buried her the next day. Father John took her to church late on August 8, after a kind pediatrician, Dr. Fenn, came to our house to pronounce her dead and give her an official diagnosis. Parishioners read psalms over Mary Rose's body and the next day we went to the cemetery. My milk was about to come in. I was about to die from grief, only I did not die. The postpartum period with the hormones raging and no baby were awful.

I worked through the difficult first year facing various milestones. Halloween. Thanksgiving. Christmas. My son's third birthday. The anniversary of the ultrasound in March. Easter which we Orthodox Christians call Pascha. Then my birthday, and I was pregnant. Having our daughter's one-year memorial service at church after a miscarriage was even more painful. Another loss. The second miscarriage in October before the second round of holidays without Mary Rose sent me into a tailspin. I felt like a failure. What if my body could no longer make healthy babies?

When I got Mary Rose's diagnosis, I vowed not to become bitter and to do right by her. I treated her pregnancy the same as my son's, though she was not expected to live. That meant not

3

taking medicine and eating healthy, though I wanted to die from my grief. Out of this life-changing experience I shifted the focus of my writing career to writing about the pregnancy and the miscarriages. I launched a blog to support bereaved mothers. Our culture does not give us space to grieve publicly. I am writing to change that. We have a right to cry and mourn our babies and pregnancies. It is so important that we support each other in a world that tells us that one child can replace another.

Given the circumstances of my life, I am doing well. Perhaps I am even thriving, though I have little patience for people's hurtful words. Why do people defend the ones who use insensitive words? "They mean well," people tell me. I am on a crusade to support others, to offer messages on Facebook to women going through similar circumstances, to send a card to a mother who has miscarried her first child, to write another blog post to offer a little bit of comfort. When I speak about my book, *Walking the Labyrinth of My Heart: A Journey of Pregnancy, Grief and Infant Death,* I will address community or the lack thereof. I want to invite people to sit with each other in the discomfort of grief and not say anything except "I am here." Can we accept pregnancy, infant loss, and the death of our loved ones as a normal and natural part of life instead of fighting death and shunning the bereaved? It is my hope that future generations of women going through such losses will be supported and loved in their grief.

*

LINDA BATEMAN GOMEZ
Linda's 8-week-old son Chad
died in 1986 from SIDS

The loss of a child, and the grief that accompanies it, has such a deep implanted space in your brain, it's almost as if that space is reserved for it. There is no other memory that has such a dedicated place to allow us in a split second to smell, feel, and relive that time again so vividly...and so painfully.

In 1986 I was pregnant with my third child, I had two beautiful, healthy little girls ages two and four. Life was wonderful! I was married to the love of my life, a young handsome doctor, and surrounded by wonderful family and friends. I was a stay-at-home mom living my dream of being a mother. It was the only thing in my life I ever really wanted to be and the only thing I ever thought I was good at.

Chad Ernest Gomez was born on June 16, a beautiful boy. Our life was truly magical and our family was complete! Chad was healthy in every way. He was born on time, had great Apgar scores and his well-baby visits were perfect! I nursed him as I had done with my girls, he latched on early and all seemed to be going smoothly. He was such a sweet baby, and had already started smiling, especially at his giggling older sisters.

The weeks that followed were so much fun! Nothing excites two little girls like a baby brother. June in Arizona is hot, so they had lots of indoor playtime together. Grandparents came to visit and the house was filled with love and family.

At about six weeks old I was nursing Chad when he did something odd, I remember it as if it was yesterday. While nursing, he pulled away as if to breathe. His nose was clear so it wasn't that, but it seemed strange. It was like he needed a deep breath and once he got it he went back to nursing normally. There was no color change, he wasn't choking and it only lasted a second, but it caught my attention. Having nursed both girls for a year, I had plenty of experience breast-feeding. I nursed them in health and through colds and, while I wasn't sure why, this seemed different. The next few days everything was fine. Mindful of what happened, but with no other issues, I thought it was an isolated incident.

A week later a similar incident occurred, like Chad was trying to catch his breath. I immediately called our pediatrician and insisted something was wrong. He told me to bring him right in, which I did, it was Friday afternoon.

The doctor examined Chad and declared him the picture of health. No fever, lungs and ears were clear, he couldn't have seemed healthier. I told the doctor about the nursing incident and he said looking at Chad's weight, he suspected Chad was drinking too fast and had to pull away to swallow. He added that the appearance of needing air was probably "normal" infant apnea. My girls hadn't had that, at least I never noticed, so I didn't even know that could be normal. I left there trusting the doctor and yet there was still a little nagging feeling that something was not right. Mother's intuition perhaps.

My husband and I decided to get a second opinion. The appointment to take Chad to a different pediatrician was scheduled for Monday, but sadly we never got the chance. On Sunday morning August 10, 1986, at eight weeks old, Chad passed away in his bassinet of SIDS.

That morning and the previous week play over and over in my head. The "what if" and "if only" plague my mind. If only things had been just a little different, maybe the outcome would have changed. The manufactured guilt of a parent that we should be able to protect our child under every circumstance holds one captive as the only person to blame because who else is there but ourselves? If only I had waken Chad for a feeding before making breakfast, perhaps he would still be here, but I hadn't. After breakfast, I went to check on him, his color wasn't right, I whisked him out of that bassinet screaming for my husband, Ernie. He said he could tell by the sound of my voice that something tragic had happened, he met me in the hall and immediately started CPR.

I ran to call 911 and remember speaking clearly so they would get the address correct. It seemed like hours, but emergency workers arrived in minutes. I remember thinking, now everything would be okay. These were skilled professionals, but their equipment failed. Chad had not responded to CPR, though Ernie never stopped until help arrived. They needed to shock Chad's heart, but the paddles didn't work. They continued CPR, so I thought once they got to the hospital and had working equipment his heart would start and he would be okay, but of course by then it was too late.

The hours that followed were a fog and yet it's so clear. They brought Chad to me just like they did at birth, only this time it was so I could say goodbye. He was all swaddled up in a little hospital blanket, I sat and held him for hours.

In the weeks that followed, I'd cry until I physically couldn't cry anymore. I just wanted to die to stop the pain, life felt unbearable. My two daughters were my only reason for living. Nothing else was enough of a reason to want to live, but that mother's need to care for her children was the only thing I could focus on. The first year was the most difficult. I was learning to navigate things I had never dealt with before, like understanding the stages of grief. It was an emotional roller coaster. Sometimes well-meaning friends and family said and did things that hurt more than they helped. Getting through the holidays, Mother's Day, and especially Chad's first birthday brought such an emptiness.

My quest to find answers and get help had me talking to people, reading books and going to support groups. These led me to some realizations. If I really wanted to heal, I had to let go of constantly wondering about the breathing incidents, the emergency equipment failure, and if the timeline the morning he died would have made a difference. The truth is, not only will I never know, none of it would change anything now. I had to move forward and let go of the "what ifs."

Then, I met a mother who also lost her baby to SIDS. She told me that in fact life does go on and the pain would get better and that one day I would be happy again. She was right. I came to understand that the horrendous pain of my broken heart may never be whole again, after all, it is missing a piece. Yet there was a light at the end of that long dark tunnel. I now have five living children and two (almost three) beautiful grandchildren. So yes, it does get better, much better. Life is good.

*

KARI BROWN
Kari's 2-year-old daughter Dominique (Deedee)
died in 2014 from obstructive sleep apnea

Dominique Faith was born two months early as a late Christmas gift on December 28, 2011. She weighed only three pounds ten ounces. We fell in love with her immediately. Deedee stayed in the NICU for four months, undergoing battles with viruses and subsequent surgeries to help her survive. She eventually was discharged from the NICU on May 3, a day after Brandon's (my fiancé, her father) birthday.

Deedee struggled to eat and speak but picked up her own talents in other ways. She communicated through American Sign Language since she was hard of hearing like myself. Brandon is also deaf, so we were elated to see that Deedee was comfortable with signing as the means of communication. Every night, Deedee would have to sleep at an angle because she had obstructive sleep apnea. I always worried that she would somehow pass away during the night because her airway became constricted. Our worries faded away as her survival rate increased. We fell so much in love with this bundle of joy that I decided to stay home and provide all her care, since she needed extra attention. We still didn't feel right for Dominique to be sleeping in her own bed with all the problems she had, so we had her sleep with us, in the middle.

One morning, while Brandon and Dominique were still asleep, I woke up and noticed that Deedee was breathing funny. I woke up Brandon, we both checked Deedee and thought she was okay. Brandon returned to sleep, and I got up to make coffee. As I was putting away Deedee's toys in her bedroom, she got down from bed and ran toward me with her little hands around her fragile neck. Her precious face was turning blue, and she attempted to cry, but nothing was coming out of her mouth. When I bent down to pick her up, she collapsed.

It felt as my heart stopped beating for that whole day when she collapsed. I ran over to Brandon with her in my arms and woke him up. We both laid her down and attempted CPR. Nothing was working. We screamed her name, we cried out loud, we called 911. but nothing was bringing her back. And then Deedee took one last attempt to breathe, and stopped. It felt like I could feel her soul leaving her body. Like she was already gone. I couldn't accept that, I couldn't comprehend that. I needed her and she needed me. She was my world, the light of my life, the reason to live.

The ride in the ambulance to the hospital felt like we were going five miles per hour. The EMT driver attempted to keep me calm, but something was telling me that she was already gone. That she would never come back into my arms again. We arrived at the hospital, but the nurses kept us at a distance. Brandon sat down in a chair because he felt sick, crying and pleading. I never felt so numb, wailing, screaming for my baby to come back to me. After some time, one of the nurses came over to us with tears in her eyes. Right then and there, I knew our baby Dominique was forever gone. I disagreed, I denied the fact that she was gone. I begged the nurse to do something, anything to save her. The nurse couldn't respond, but offered to let us hold Dominique one last time. We held her. And cried, cried and cried. I kept begging Dominique to please wake up and come back to us. But she never did.

An autopsy later revealed that she had suffered from a constricted airway. Our biggest fear actually came true. I blamed myself for not doing more for Deedee, for not disagreeing with the doctors and taking action when I knew something was still wrong. For not waking up Dominique that morning when she was breathing funny.

*

MARY LEE CLAFLIN
Mary Lee's 2-month-old grandson Lane
died in 1998 from carbon monoxide poisoning

In early 1997, I was told by my son and daughter-in-law that I was going to be a grandmother in October. I was not like most parents that wanted their children to have a grandbaby. I was not ready for that chapter in my life. My son had told his sister he was worried that I showed no excitement about the baby.

On the morning of October 21, my son called to say that the baby was coming. I left work and drove to the hospital. My son came out to the waiting room to tell me it would not be long. They already knew it would be a boy. My daughter-in-law Charmayne named the baby Lane Edward after her father. Once we were allowed in the room they gave me the baby to hold. All at once he took over my heart. I fell in love with this beautiful baby, the same one I was not excited about.

Since my son lived near me, I would leave from work every day at 4:30 p.m. and head over to their house to help with the baby. When I appeared at the door they would hand Lane to me and he became mine. I changed his diapers, fed him and rocked him to sleep. This went on for almost two months. My love grew bigger and bigger for this baby.

It was now January 1998, and time for my daughter-in-law to go back to work. They did not want to place Lane in a nursery and, since I worked at a church, they asked if I knew anyone who kept children in their home. I knew a lady in the choir who had her grandson in a friend's home. That lady gave me a name and number and I passed it on to my son.

They met with the lady who just so happened to live around the corner from me and near the church. She told my son she only kept one infant at a time and several toddlers. She was willing to keep Lane. She answered all the questions that they asked of her, including whether she had a license to keep children in her home.

10

If you keep more than a certain number of children, you must have a license and your home must be inspected. The kids were happy with this lady.

On Monday, January 5, they dropped Lane at the sitter's. My daughter-in-law called me late morning asking if I could run over on my lunch hour and check on Lane. New mothers hate leaving their babies in the beginning. I went over to the sitter's house and met her. I was on the list to pick Lane up if needed. He was sleeping in his infant seat on the sofa so I did not wake him, and went back to work.

That night my daughter-in-law called me and asked if Lane seemed okay when I saw him. I said yes but that he was sleeping when I got there. She was worried that the baby did not seem okay but could not put her finger on it.

On January 6, they dropped Lane off again and went to work. At 4 p.m. that afternoon they received a call from the sitter saying Lane was not breathing. My daughter-in-law Charmayne arrived and saw nothing but ambulances, fire trucks and police cars blocking the street. They rushed Lane to the nearest hospital. That night the rain poured down for hours. The hospital wanted to have Lane airlifted to the medical center where he could get specialized care but rain prohibited the helicopter to fly, so they sent him by ambulance.

Once we got to the hospital they let us see Lane for a few minutes. He was hooked up to a machine that was keeping him alive. I called a dear friend as well as my pastor and they came to be with us. We all spent the entire night just waiting. Charmayne wanted Lane baptized before they pronounced him dead. I had my two pastors to perform this act. As the pastor sprinkled water on his head he repeated these words that were spoken at Jesus' baptism, "This is my beloved son, in whom I am well pleased."

Finally on the morning of January 7, the doctors told us there was no brain activity; we needed to decide about turning off the machine. I was given one last time to hold my grandbaby. He was so warm yet lifeless, he looked like he was sleeping. Once the machine was turned off, he made no sound for he had already died.

Seeing a baby who lived two months, two weeks and two days lay in a casket is heart-wrenching. The church was packed for his service. We were all just devastated. How were we to go on without this baby in our lives? This same baby that I was once not excited about but fell in love with?

It turned out that the sitter did not have a license to keep children, and no inspection was ever done. She had placed Lane in the upstairs bedroom to nap and he died from carbon monoxide poisoning. It only affected him because he was so young, and the only one upstairs. For seventeen years I carried the burden of guilt that had I not recommended this lady, Lane might still be alive. It was my fault. Then a great therapist told me it was not guilt I was feeling, but regret. For Lane's eighteenth birthday I only felt regret. Even though he was in our life for a short time, he was loved greatly and never forgotten.

*

ANNAH ELIZABETH
Annah Elizabeth's son Gavin Michael aspirated on his meconium during delivery in 1990 and died 26 minutes following his birth

I recall three distinct childhood memories: I wanted to change the world, to end hate, injustice and suffering. I dreamt of being a writer. I wanted one day to be a mom, but not an old mom, so I was going to have those babies before I turned thirty.

Like most teenagers, I experienced the normal worries about not being good enough, not smart enough and not pretty enough. And like many a teenager, though most people never knew how I felt on the inside, I struggled to fit in. I graduated high school, went to college, found a job and met a boy.

A whirlwind romance later, I found myself five hundred miles away in another state with a new job and a failed relationship. My parents offered to come move me back home, but for some unknown reason, I chose to stay in this new town. Initially, I stayed because I hoped that beau and I would work things out, but one day I woke up and realized I deserved so much more than the manipulation he'd offered. Afterward? I didn't give it a thought until years later. You see, I never believed in fate or destiny, and then a man came to fix the broken lock on my front door and my life was forever changed.

That handyman and I quickly became friends. Nearly four months later we went out on our first date and four years after that we were newly married and expecting our first child. I was twenty-six-years-old and life was rolling along right according to my master plan. That pregnancy progressed without so much as a hiccup and I worked right up until the day before I delivered.

We thought we'd prepared for everything. We'd read parenting books, followed prenatal advice and I'd swallowed those enormous vitamins. We'd baby-proofed the house, prepared the nursery, pre-washed the clothing, sterilized the baby's things, picked out names and attended Lamaze classes. In one of our later birthing classes, the instructor addressed the group like this: "I know you're all in happy places with even happier times ahead, but I want you to think about something. What would you do if something happened to the baby? I know it's not anything you want to think about, but you really should spend a minute or two discussing it." "What would you do if something happened to the baby," I asked Warren on the way home that night.

"I don't know. You?" he replied. "I don't know, either," I responded. We didn't talk about it again. Until we had to.

On May 11, 1990, my labor progressed exactly as all the doctors and books had said it would. Shortly after the nurse hooked me up to the monitors, all of that changed. An emergency cesarean section later, doctors discovered that my son had aspirated on his meconium, the baby's first stool. While Warren sat in the waiting room and I lay asleep under anesthesia, a medical team worked to save my son's life. Gavin Michael, unable to overcome his circumstances, died twenty-six minutes after he quietly entered this world.

Those early days, weeks and months are a blur, but I do remember one thing clearly. Even in those earliest mourning days as I recovered in the hospital, I knew I didn't want to spend a lifetime grieving my son. I didn't know what that meant, what it looked like on the other side, or how I was ever going to get there, but I knew what I didn't want.

The casseroles dried out. The well of visitors and sympathy cards dried up. I grieved. I cried. I smiled when I saw a rainbow. I felt like I had betrayed my son's memory. I returned to work. I worried I would forget my child. I pleaded with the universe for understanding. I asked questions. I found a few answers. I blamed myself.

I'd always known I was going to be a mom, so the second the doctor gave Warren and me the go-ahead, we began trying to conceive. I'm one of those "Fertile Myrtles." I've always joked that all Warren had to do was unzip his pants and, Voila! I was pregnant. Almost eight weeks into that next pregnancy, I miscarried. I went into an emotional tailspin. I questioned God, my own spirituality, my role as a woman, a mother, a wife and my place on Earth. And I stayed true to my plan. I was going to be a mom, one way or another. Warren and I signed on and began the lengthy, tedious process of becoming foster parents. When my obstetrician gave us the green light, well, you know, our bedroom came alive again.

Flash forward seven years, I'd had two more complicated but successful pregnancies, a second miscarriage, had spent six weeks in a psyche ward for severe depression, and was seven months pregnant when I discovered that my best friend and my husband were having an affair.

I sat slumped in a heap against my washing machine for hours. This is what I later wrote about that morning. "Every piece of hope I'd ever held on to before had just been shredded. My faith in people, my trust; my belief in God, in dignity--every spiritual, emotional, social, physical, and academic part of me lay in a heap to be tossed out with the garbage. It never made it to the garbage. I recycled it instead."

The part of me that knew I didn't want to spend a lifetime in mourning urged me to get up off that floor and it screamed at me to do something. I eventually did. I pulled myself up to a standing position and reached out, once again, for help.

All those unanswered questions I'd ignored when work, diapers, preschool, scouts, and sports got in the way came back with a vengeance. I knew that if I were to get to the other side, I had to give those queries serious attention and I had to find answers.

One main question stood above the rest. How can some people survive death or destruction or disease and go on to live happy, healthy lives, while others of similar circumstance succumb to despair or, worse, drugs or suicide, and are forever held back from living their best lives? These are some of the realizations I discovered: Grief encompasses much more than death.

Though we have countless resources to help us with our bereavement, we have little other than platitude to guide us once we decide our grief is no longer serving us a purpose. We need to *add* the healing piece. Healing doesn't mean that what happened is okay; rather it means that we can be okay in the face of it. We're all born with everything we need to heal. Though the details of our resources and circumstances are different for each of us, the crux of the matter is the same: We've all encountered some event that has led to grief which wants to be healed. And right next door are neighbors who are also suffering and allies who can help us on our own journey to healing.

*

RENEE FORD-ROMERO
Renee's son Diego was stillborn due
to an undiagnosed cardiac fibroma in 2014

In 2013 we were *very* surprised to find out we were pregnant. At the time, our daughter was five and it took us eight years to have her. Joy, elation, euphoria, there aren't enough synonyms to describe how we were feeling. Mostly though, so grateful for a second chance at a miracle. I have Polycystic Ovarian Syndrome which causes all sorts of interesting imbalances and pretty much prevents ovulation. Everything was going well with the pregnancy but we lost our baby girl in July. I had just gotten over Strep throat, had a pretty high fever and a urinary tract infection. Of course I blamed myself for the loss (that's what I do). If I had washed my hands more……no amount of attempted convincing by my doctor worked. An unexplained second trimester miscarriage, we were devastated and clung to each other and to our faith.

Shortly after, my husband and I accepted an invitation by our pastor to host a small group bible study in our home but right before it started I miscarried again. I didn't even know I was pregnant, I didn't know you could get pregnant so quickly after a loss. Again, we had that baby tested for genetic disorders and everything came back perfect, another unexplained loss.

Although we were grieving these babies, we remained very excited about serving God through our small group and we knew God would bless us for keeping our commitment. I don't know about you but the enemy lies to me; he says there's too much going on, you're not qualified, your house isn't big enough, and nobody's going to show up. But like I said, lies! The relationships we made in our small group enriched our lives greatly. I found so much freedom in building relationships with my family in Christ! We also started ministering to the homeless (very healing for me) and teaching in children's ministry.

We were absolutely shocked to find out in December I was pregnant again. I thought okay, third time's the charm, life is awesome, and we're getting off this emotional rollercoaster. However, my son Diego Ramon Romero was stillborn on May 6, 2014. I was in labor nine hours, the entire time knowing he'd never take a breath on this side of Heaven. He was absolutely beautiful. I studied him, every detail and have managed to tuck away into my heart every feature of his beautiful face, his teeny tiny hands, and his perfect toes. I've tucked it away and allow myself to visit once in a while. It keeps us safe, "us" meaning myself and the memory of him. To visit too often would be to relive grief and pain so indescribable that anyone who has not held a lifeless child could never possibly understand.

I couldn't force a smile for so long, I was so angry! My husband and I were serving faithfully, we were running full speed toward Jesus and had the rug pulled out from under us. This time though, we got our answers. Not another unexplained loss. The autopsy showed a cardiac fibroma, a tumor in Diego's heart that was either missed on a previous ultrasound or grew very quickly. We've lost another pregnancy since, twins on August 7, because of an infection caused by tissue retained during the birth of Diego. Each loss uniquely horrifying but even in my grief I can hear God, I can see His hand in everything.

*

NEISHA HART
Neisha's 6-month-old daughter
Brimley died in 2015 to SUID

On June 25, 2014, we welcomed a beautiful little baby into our family by the name of Brimley Shyanne Barks. She had the smile of an angel from the very start. It didn't matter who you were, she always flashed a grinning smile with love.

My pregnancy was the typical textbook pregnancy, once we had found out that is. I was in my junior year of college and

17

finishing up the last of my classes before my year-long internship started. I had gone to the campus health clinic to get a refill on a prescription I had ran out of. The nurse was asking all the normal questions and then she got to one, when was your last period? I looked over at Brad, with whom I had been for over two years, and kind of gave him a blank stare. I responded with, "Well, it's been a couple of months now that I think of it." She mentioned that when we got a chance, I should take a home pregnancy test just to check.

It seemed like I couldn't get home fast enough. Even though pregnancy wasn't in our plan, I happened to have a test at home. I jolted through the door to take it. Two lines showed up as dark as could be before the test was even finished. Brad and I once again gave each other that blank stare. We were going to be parents.

Flash forward thirty weeks, I was thirty-eight weeks pregnant and ready for my baby girl to be here. We got to the hospital late Tuesday night for induction to start. By noon the next day, after hours of agonizing pain, I was finally dilated enough for the doctor to break my water. Every hour the doctor would be in to check progress, which was slowly and surely getting nowhere! At 6 p.m. that night it was decided, and a cesarean section it was.

The next five hours seemed to be kind of a blur to me. Brad was changing into his scrubs and booties while I was in the OR getting prepped for surgery. Over the next forty-five minutes, the anesthesiologist would push more and more needles into my back at the request of me. I wanted Brad to be there with me while our precious child was being born. The anesthesiologist stopped four times and said that he couldn't find a place for a spinal, and each time I would beg him to try just one more time. Finally, enough was enough. I had to be put under general anesthesia, and the normal cesarean section was now an emergency one. After the anesthetic is administered into the body, doctors have ninety seconds to get the baby out before the anesthesia takes over their body too. Our baby had arrived at 8:35 p.m., happy and healthy.

Our baby girl's favorite things to do were smile and laugh at everyone who walked by, playing fetch with her favorite ball with grandpa, playing with her feet, and as always listening to music and dancing with daddy. She loved spending time with mommy and her grandmas, and any kind of music. Brimley and her Aunt Tiffany had an amazing bond that words couldn't even begin to describe. To this day, it still amazes me when I think about it.

On January 9, 2015, our world came to a screeching halt. I went into the nursery that morning around 9 a.m. to get my little girl up. When I went in and saw her face, I knew instantly something was seriously wrong. Her eyes were slightly open and her lips were blue. Brad had fallen asleep on the couch that night, and I ran to where he was and screamed, "Brimley isn't breathing!" I grabbed her from the crib and brought her out to the living room and called 911. As the phone was ringing instincts kicked in to unzip her sleeper and get ready to start CPR. With the help of the 911 dispatcher both Brad and I alternated compressions and breaths until paramedics arrived. They did all they could but unfortunately without knowing how long she hadn't been breathing, it was just too late.

Looking back that whole day is just a blurry nightmare. Family arrived at the house to try and comfort and console one another, but what was going to change the fact that we had just lost our perfectly healthy baby girl? Nothing. Brimley lets us know that she is safe and happy where she is, but nothing will heal the feeling of loneliness and heartbreak.

The funeral director let us do what we thought was the unthinkable after the funeral service had ended. We got to swaddle our little girl up just like we had every night before, in her favorite blanket that one of her great-grandmothers had made her. We got time to hold her and kiss her and tell her everything would be all right. We told her she would never have to be scared, and there were family members waiting for her who would keep her safe. My angel's smile will never be forgotten.

The one thing that hurts the most is that we don't have answers about why this nightmare happened. Maybe someday we will, but for right now we just keep asking why her? Why us?

Just over three months had passed and I got the call I had been waiting for. Brimley's death certificate had arrived. That same day we went and got it, ultimately to see if the examiners had found a cause of death. As our gut had been telling us, we didn't....the cause of death was labeled SUID, Sudden Unexpected Infant Death.

We did research upon research to try and get answers. What we found was the death certificate is labeled this when a cause of death cannot be determined. The very next day I called the medical examiner's office to request a copy of the autopsy. When we got it, it just told us what we had known. She was healthy. Never once had she been sick, not even a common cold and there were no answers of what had happened.

The impact that our baby had on our lives was in every way possible. She taught us all how to love a little harder, smile a little longer, and to laugh a little more. She taught us not to worry about the little things but to look at the bigger picture. She taught us not to pass judgment on others, not to argue about the petty stuff, and that even when the days seem the darkest the light will indeed shine again!

Brimley will always be my gift! I am so beyond blessed to be able to be her mommy and have the amount of time I did with her. I was lucky enough to be able to have known her nine months, before anyone else, while she was growing inside me. Every so often I still seem to get "phantom kicks" inside my belly, and it just reminds me how blessed I was that I got to call her mine! Those are truly memories that I can never forget.

*

BELINDA LUNA
Belinda's full-term baby Elijah
died in utero in 2012 from trisomy 18

I remember like it was yesterday. I had been going through a lot of ups and downs with my sons' father. We were on again off again. He struggled with addiction and after our first son was born, he changed and was never really the same. I guess you could say I was in an abusive relationship. I ended up pregnant in 2012, when our first son was two and I was happy when I found out I was pregnant but also very worried for some reason.

The first few months I was in and out of the hospital. I always felt like something just wasn't right. I had never felt that way with any of my other pregnancies. I was under so much stress and was preparing myself to raise both my sons on my own. On October 12, 2012, I went in for an ultrasound and to determine the sex of my angel. But that wasn't the only news I received. I was told that my son was showing signs of spina bifida. I couldn't speak, I was frozen. It all seemed surreal.

I was sent to San Francisco for a level II ultrasound. That's the day I was told my son was paralyzed from the waist down, that he had severe clubbed feet and a small brain hemorrhage. They performed an amniocentesis and I traveled home waiting for a phone call. A genetic specialist explained that what we didn't want to see was an extra chromosome on the 13 or 18 because that would mean Elijah had Trisomy 13 or 18.

Two days later I got the call and she told me that my son had thirty-nine out of forty-six abnormal chromosomes. Wow...I was in pure shock. I said, "Thank you," and hung the phone up. I was numb. I couldn't cry or even be mad. Nothing came out.

I spent the rest of that month researching trisomy 18. Elijah had full trisomy 18! Most males with the disease succumb in the womb just as Elijah did. I chose not to hold my son or look at his face; I didn't want that to be the one and only image of my baby. I was

21

already traumatized in a way that I could never put into words. On December 5, 2012, my full-term son was born sleeping. The past almost three years have been filled with ups and downs and questions like what if I had done this or that differently.

Grief is such a complex thing and we all experience it differently except for the immense pain and heartache we all feel. That is hard for me to express sometimes, actually most the time. I don't talk too much about it for fear of making others uncomfortable. I do know one thing for sure: it has changed me forever. I am just different and a lot of people don't understand. I've lost friends along the way. It's sad but I try every day to find my lesson in such a huge loss. That's my test I think, trying to extract the good out of a tragic circumstance. I have to have faith that there is something big for me to learn, I just don't know what that is yet.

*

MELISSA MEAD
Melissa's 13-month-old son
William died in 2014 from sepsis

William, or Grumpus as he was affectionately known to us, was a miracle that we never thought possible. After many medical complications, nine operations, removal of one whole ovary and half of the other, William arrived on my birthday: November 27, 2013, born at the same time his father Paul was born.

William was the most delightful baby, he was perfect and more than we could have ever have dreamed of. William flourished into a calm and happy baby who never failed to light a room up with his smile and infectious laugh. Every day was a blessing. I would often find myself sitting and watching William, in total disbelief that he was actually mine.

William started nursery when he was ten months old and proved to be an intelligent, considerate child. He was developing exceptionally well. Shortly after starting nursery William felt poorly at the end of September 2014 with scarlet fever. Just a few days after this he developed a chesty cough. After several trips to the doctors, we were assured that William's cough was a normal "nursery" cough. The cough persisted over the coming weeks and then William began to vomit five to six times a day. Again, we took him to the doctors several times, and we were once again reassured this was normal. William learnt how to live with his cough, though it hindered his energy levels and affected his eating.

We celebrated our birthdays together, William had a little party with a beautiful cake. This would prove to be his first and last birthday. A couple of days after his first birthday he took his first independent steps, I was elated.

The cough continued to plague him and when William spiked a temperature of 40.1 Celsius, we rushed him to an emergency appointment, only to be told that he had a virus. We were to give him paracetamol and fluids. Over the next twenty-four hours William deteriorated and I called 111 to seek advice and was told it wasn't an emergency. I later spoke to another doctor who assured us William was suffering from a virus, and that bed rest and fluids were the best thing for him.

After checking on William several times during the night, I went to wake him on the morning of Sunday, December 14. William had blackout blinds in his nursery so I couldn't see very well. I leant into his cot and stroked his cheek and he didn't stir. I knelt down and stroked his arm through the bars of his cot, I rubbed his side and he was stiff. I threw the curtains open to find him passed away. I knew he was gone. He was cold and stiff, his eyes staring straight through me. I immediately called 999 and started CPR but there was nothing I or the paramedics could do. He was gone. My world ended in that moment.

Weeks later after a postmortem it was established that William had in fact been suffering with pneumonia, fluid had built up in his lung cavity causing empyema which seeped into his bloodstream and caused sepsis. After an inquest, it was established that William's life could have been saved even as late as the evening before his death. This, if it's at all possible, makes the pain worse, knowing that William died needlessly. The ensuing months have been torturous and continue to be.

*

TAMARA NOVOTNY-KAUP
Tamara's 25-day-old daughter
Taylor Reanne died in 1995 of streptococcus

After trying to get pregnant multiple times, I'd just about given up. Oh, I could GET pregnant, I just couldn't STAY pregnant. I have been pregnant a total of eight times between 1982 and 2000, gave birth four times, but it seems like it took doctors almost eighteen years to come to the conclusion that I might have had an incompetent cervix.

It was around the beginning of June 1994 when I came home from the doctor's office with a BIG positive written in red on my medical receipt. I'm extra excited this time and I can't wait for my husband to either call home or come home – but knowing he just left for work he wasn't due to come home until the next morning. I was on dayshift and he was on graveyard, so I knew it was going to make me crazy not being able to tell him right away! We followed doctor's orders explicitly, including walking around the block, eating healthy and getting plenty of sleep. My doctor always said, "Just when you think you're getting enough sleep – get another hour." I was pretty careful to pack a lunch for work, or at least choose to eat somewhere well known.

One morning the food list was going around the dispatch floor and everyone was raving about this particular restaurant's chicken-fried steak. Although I'd never eaten there before, it was frequented by our center. So I ordered it and ate about half. I began feeling bloated so I stopped eating it. Not thinking much about "why," I just put it in the refrigerator for later. I remember taking it home and it smelled odd when I reheated it, so I just threw it in the trash.

Later that evening I had to call into my work to get the fire department to come check my vital signs, as I knew I had food poisoning. I was up all night long, and had vomited so violently all the blood vessels on the surface of my face had ruptured and my eyes were bloodshot. The medics told me to keep drinking water so I didn't get dehydrated. I did that but just kept vomiting. When I had reached a calm, I called my husband to come home and he took me to the hospital. I was there for a little more than an hour while they rehydrated me. They gave me the okay to go home and rest, so I did just that. My husband said I didn't move until that next evening!

Halloween and Thanksgiving came and went, and our lives seemed to be back on track. We were getting ready for Christmas and the kids, then five and seven years-old, were excited for their upcoming holiday vacation. I was six months pregnant by this time when on the morning of December 11, I woke up with slight cramping and when I got out of bed, my water broke - or so I thought, as there wasn't much fluid. Odd, I remembered a more flood-like experience before. I decided it was my imagination, and could just sit down and get ready for work as I contemplated the consequences. It was my "Friday" at work, and the supervisors are especially hard on people on their Mondays and Fridays. Added to that fact was that we were going live on a new phone system that same day. They had already announced that they'd need all hands on deck, so I continued to get ready for work.

As I drove through the gate and parked the car, I felt a strong urge to use the restroom. I sat still in the car for a moment to see if the feeling would pass, as I had to walk past the off-going shift of people just to get to the facility in the building. Just as I walked into the bathroom, a gush of water flowed down my legs. I remember

25

thanking God for dressing in my leggings and a long sweater that day. I walked into the room where I worked and my supervisor asked how I was doing. I opened my sweater to reveal the obvious evidence of my water breaking. She didn't waste any time and immediately took me to the hospital I had previously registered at, in Upland which was a twenty to twenty-five-minute drive away.

As I walked in through the maternity door, I remember hearing my supervisor tell the nurse that my water broke. The rest is a fog though I recall laying on a hospital bed with my supervisor sitting in a chair next to me. She said she was going to sit there until my husband arrived. I felt badly, as my husband had to drive in traffic and he took over an hour to arrive. Bless her heart, she insisted on sitting in that uncomfortable chair so I wouldn't be alone.

According to the doctors and nurses, I was not allowed to get out of that bed for any reason until I had my baby. This was night one of four unbearably uncomfortable days and nights. I stayed in bed, watched TV, tried sleeping and had to use bed pans! I would just about lose my mind and then had to remember why I was there and tell myself it would all be worth it once I got to meet my little doll-faced angel.

On the afternoon of December 14, I became unusually bloated and my back was hurting much more than usual. I told the nurse that I might be in labor and she checked and sure enough I was. Holy cow, I wasn't supposed to deliver for another three months! Now what? Well, they wheeled me in to Labor & Delivery and slathered my stomach with gel to check on the baby. The machine wasn't working, so they had to get another one. All the while I'm propped up, legs spread wide open, gel all over my belly with techs, nurses, aides and a doctor waiting on another machine. Yep—yikes!

By now my mother and husband have been called and are on their way to the hospital. Before the machine gets wheeled into the room – out popped my newborn baby. I don't hear any crying and as I look around, a nurse and another doctor are in the room rushing around and immediately take off with the baby. I don't know if it's a boy or a girl at this point. I was cleaned up and wheeled into a different area of the maternity ward where I was met by my doctor and husband. It was then that we were told we had a daughter and that we all had a very long road ahead of us. Because she was premature, she didn't have very strong lungs plus she had some obvious underdevelopment. The doctor took us to the NICU to see her. She was in a warming bed, had tubes connected all over, but we could touch her and talk to her. The doctor then said that our baby girl had had too much stimulation for one day. We went back to my room and all I could do was cry. My mom and grandmother were there by now and did their best to keep my spirits up.

I was discharged home without my baby girl, and the days remain a blur. Although I have a daily diary, it doesn't make sense to anyone else but my husband and I at this point. I just remember feeling like I was not doing enough for my baby, so I made sure to get to the hospital each and every day. I was only able to touch her a handful of times and hold her once while she was still alive. She did well when I held her, yet they wouldn't let me do so any more than that one time. It was very confusing. When a baby is born, nurturing is HUGE, and we were BOTH denied that opportunity.

About a week before we lost Taylor, she found out she had contracted a bacterial infection. She was given antibiotics to help her fight it, but she was already overmedicated with steroids and vitamins so they weren't sure how she could handle more. Taylor passed away on a Sunday evening, January 8, 1995, at 6:06 p.m. They said she died from being so weak; she had been fighting to grow, fighting to stay alive and fight off other airborne illnesses that can be contracted while in a neonatal unit.

My baby girl died at twenty-five days old to Strep bacteria. To this day, I still deliberate whether there was something I should have or could have done differently. I have huge guilt thinking I am the one who failed our baby. I know the cause of death is premature birth associated with a horrible bacterial virus, but why was she premature? Why won't anyone tell me? I was hurting so badly, I couldn't think straight. I had five and seven-year-old children, a husband, a mother, grandmother, aunts, in-laws and friends all around and I couldn't see them.

After our baby's funeral and over the years since that windy January afternoon in 1995, I went from visiting her gravesite every month, to visiting just during holidays and then, after my mother passed away and I needed to attend to my grandmother, I have only made it around Christmas — and I have missed two Christmases now. I have heard that funerals and visiting burial sites is for the living, and I do believe it makes me feel better when I go, but I also feel it's a duty. I owe the one I'm visiting since I am still alive. So to avoid that feeling, I tend to avoid the entire visit – then feel guilty. The cycle has been going on for so long that I've just adjusted.

If I had one thing to take away from this entire experience, it would be support. Trust your support system! I had so many people around me helping me, willing to do so much for me and I was too proud, too ashamed and naïve that I didn't allow anyone "in" for quite a while. I had to go back to work, not after a normal maternity leave, but I gave birth and buried my baby and had nothing but guilt to show for it. No one knew how to approach me. No one knew what they could or couldn't say that may or may not have hurt me. The awkwardness on all ends was emotionally depleting. I think having a strong support system around is most important, as it took me a long time to snap out of my "cloud" of depression but once I did I was able to SEE the support and work my way through our loss.

Don't get me wrong, I still cry when I think of how much we all miss out not having Taylor in our lives. I look at our fourteen-year-old daughter now and wish I could have had more time, as I'm sure they'd look alike, sound alike and I picture their laughs being alike. We also include Taylor in every bit of our lives, as if she was with us in the physical. I have her stuffed animals in my room, I make sure her ornaments make it on our tree each year. I do try to get up to her gravesite – at least around the holidays. My cousin designed her marker and also made us a copy to keep with us and we have it hung on our wall. Taylor would be twenty-one years-old this December, so that's hopefully the last "what if" memory I will have to get past. I used to just cry when I thought of her, I now am finally able to smile with those tears.

*

SUSAN WILLIAMS
Susan's 2-month-old son
Tony died in 1987 from SIDS

It was one week before Holy Week in March 1987. My maternity leave was coming to an end, and I needed to see what my substitute teacher had covered, and where I needed to start when I returned to work. I had one week left with my two sons before I returned back to school. It would be so nice to celebrate Easter with two babies. Zach was two, and Tony was two months old. The grandparents were so excited to have the kids come and share the holiday with them.

Tuesday would be a perfect day to drop the children off at their new sitter, and catch up on what was going on in my music classroom. The sitter lived about two miles from me. She was perfect. She had other children who were the same age as Zach. The only problem I had was getting an appropriate bed for Tony to sleep in at her house, as she did not have a crib. When I left both boys in the morning, Zach was crying but the baby was fine. I wasn't worried. I would be back around noon. When I got to school I remember being in the teachers' lounge and my principal told me to grab the phone. He said it was an emergency. Immediately my babysitter told me not to "freak out." Now I knew I would! I thought it must be Zachary, because he was crying when I left. She said the baby is in ER, and I need to get there as fast as I can. I was thirty minutes away from the hospital.

When I arrived at the hospital, they immediately put me in a room where my babysitter was sitting and crying her eyes out. She was totally in shock. She told me she had laid the baby down on her waterbed, and when she checked on him he wasn't breathing. Within five minutes of being in the room, a doctor came in to tell both of us that the baby had died. Both of us just lost it. She screamed and screamed. I asked for a bedpan because I was going to throw up.

I really don't remember when she left, but I was left alone with a social worker. He gave me a phone and helped me place calls to my parents, and to my husband. My husband was more than an hour away. My parents were also an hour away. Miraculously, the priest from my parish was on his way. Within ten minutes he walked me outside and spoke about his mother who had ten children and lost one in infancy. She never stopped loving that child. That brought me a lot of comfort for some reason. He never said anything about God. He shared his experience that he had with his mother.

When my husband and parents came, we all embraced and went to see Tony. I wanted to hold him and so did Stu. My parents did the same. I was amazed that my parents were able to hold their dead grandchild, but they did. Those memories are the most horrible to bear as a mother and a daughter. Holding your lifeless child when he was a healthy baby hours ago is beyond understanding. Seeing your mom and dad hold their dead grandchild sucked every tear I had out of my eyes.

After we had all held the baby, the nurses had a prescription for me to take if I needed it. I remember saying, "Absolutely not!" I knew I would take it. I knew I did not want anything that I could take that would kill me in my house. I knew I wanted to die. That feeling did not leave me for many months. I truly wanted to die. The only reason I would not allow myself to abuse drugs or alcohol was for my parents, my son and my husband. I did not want them to go through losing me on top of the sorrow they were already going through. After leaving the hospital and kissing my parents, Stu and I went to the babysitter's house and picked up Zach who was still there. I can't remember too much of what happened. I know that the babysitter's husband handled a very critical emotional situation. At that moment, I knew that both of our families would never be the same.

*

Tomorrow is your birthday.
But just yesterday I could hear your voice,
smell your hair, touch your skin.
It's been five years, but the pain still runs deep.
So very, very deep.

They say the pain changes with time. It hasn't.
But I have. My coping skills are stronger. I am stronger.
I like to think I'm a better person with more compassion,
more awareness of the world outside my own.
But the pain runs deep.
So very, very deep.

The tears still fall, and from time to time
I need to retreat to The Wailing Tent
where I'm among sisters. I suppose I always will.
For the pain runs deep.
So very, very deep.

But most days the sun shines bright, and I am grateful.
Today is not one of those days, though.
I want to tell you happy birthday,
but the words just won't come.
I know I'm a few hours early anyway,
so maybe the words will come tomorrow.
Oh, the pain runs deep.
So very, very deep.

It feels like yesterday that I could hear your voice,
smell your hair, and touch your skin.
I wish it were yesterday.

LYNDA CHELDELIN FELL

*

CHAPTER TWO

THE AFTERMATH

Somehow, even in the worst of times, the tiniest fragments of good survive. – MELINA MARCHETTA

Following profound loss, the first questions we often ask ourselves are: How am I going to survive this? How can I function when I have no feeling or when those sensations are so strong they threaten to paralyze me? How can I cook and clean and cope? There we stand in the aftermath, feeling vulnerable and often ravaged with fear. How do we survive?

*

DIANNA VAGIANOS ARMENTROUT
Dianna lost her newborn baby
Mary Rose in 2014 to trisomy 18

I didn't think that I would survive the postpartum period. The milk came in the day after Mary Rose's funeral, two days after her birth and death. The pain was intense. My husband rushed back to work, while I had afterpains and dealt with the milk. I didn't know that hormones wake new mothers up at night, not the baby. I lay awake for hours each night, my eyes darting around looking for my baby. "Where is my baby," I asked again and again. My midwife said that my whole body was crying, that Mary Rose was my phantom limb. Dealing with the milk was intense and I learned a few ways to help stop it, though it took several weeks for the pain to go away. I couldn't pump and give Mary Rose's milk to another baby. I had pumped for my son who could not nurse and I had trauma around pumping. I used Sudafed, crushed cabbage leaves, ice packs, essential oil of peppermint in a carrier oil and drank lots and lots of No More Milk tea and sage tea. The postpartum period without my baby was worse than I anticipated. The grief was so physical: the soreness after labor, the new milk, the empty arms.

My hormones wanted to nurture a baby. In looking back, I coped by preparing packages for people. I sent packages to my greatest supporters during the pregnancy, such as my therapist, homeopath, midwives and doula. I gathered rose tea and candles. A book. Small things. I did this that fall and again at Christmas. Two of my poems came out in two books by Christmas, and I sent them to many people. It was a way of channeling my energy as a new mother into taking care of someone. I also put too much energy into Christmas and my son's third birthday. It was as if I was putting my love for both of my children into making my son's holidays and milestones extra special.

I wrote a lot. I worked through the workbook *Mending Invisible Wings: Healing From the Loss of Your Baby*, by Mary Burgess and Shiloh Sophia McCloud. I colored pictures, made my own drawings and paintings and wrote poems. I made one picture of Mary Rose's birth scene. I made another one with a labyrinth where the title of my blog and book came from. I cut out sympathy cards to decorate a wooden box that would hold Mary Rose's very few things. I wept. I cried. I wanted to stay on the floor and never get up. I wanted the earth to take me into her.

My son was two and a half when Mary Rose died. He, too, was processing his trauma. "Where is my sister?" he asked the day after she was born. "Where is Mary Rose?" Taking care of him and myself in our grief was difficult. I had to stay in each moment and not think ahead. I didn't let myself think "She would have been two months old." I felt Mary Rose around me, but I wanted my baby.

As a military family stationed in Norfolk, Virginia, we have no family here. My mother stayed with us for almost two months during what I now call the "Summer of Mary Rose." Mom went on family medical leave, left my father in New York, and came to take care of us. I looked to my moms' group as well as our parish to be my community, but they let me down. I attended a MOPS, Mothers of Preschoolers, meeting before the one-month anniversary of Mary Rose's birth. Initially people were kind, if a little nervous around me. But as the months went by, I felt like I was expected not to talk about Mary Rose. Of course I mentioned her every time someone asked me how many children I had. In our parish, two babies were born right after Mary Rose. The day they were baptized, I thought I would die from the pain in my heart.

Mary Rose was buried in her baptismal gown. No one ever mentioned Mary Rose. It was expected that I would buck up and move on, get over it, have another child, adopt or something. After several months of being in that church with no support, I left because I couldn't bear that the very people who sang at her funeral failed to keep her alive with me. Elizabeth McCracken is right when she says that grief lasts longer than sympathy.

*

LINDA BATEMAN GOMEZ
Linda's 8-week-old son Chad
died in 1986 from SIDS

In the hours that followed, I felt like I was in a fog and yet it's so clear. They brought the baby to me just like they do when they are born: all swaddled up in a little hospital blanket. I remember thinking that his color looked better, and I sat and held him for hours. I talked and sang to him. As odd as it sounds, while I clearly knew he was gone, as long as I was holding him, I felt like there was still hope. I really believed if I prayed hard enough, God would hear me and the baby would start to breathe again.

They finally coaxed my baby from me and Ernie led me out of the hospital in an almost zombie-like state. It was a hot August day and I didn't feel a thing, just numbness. The shock was overcome by reality when we got into the car. I remember looking out the window on the drive home realizing that life hadn't stopped for the rest of the world. Everyone was simply carrying on as normal. Shopping, driving, eating....it didn't even compute that life could go on, as my perfect world was shattered and the pain was far more than I could take. I would cry until I physically couldn't anymore and then I just wanted to die to stop the pain.

Life felt unbearable. My two daughters were my only reason for living. Not my husband, or other family, was enough of a reason to want to live, but that mother's need to care for her children was the only thing I could focus on. And so I did.

*

KARI BROWN
Kari's 2-year-old daughter Dominique (Deedee)
died in 2014 from obstructive sleep apnea

I honestly don't really remember the first few weeks. But I remember feeling physically sick. I lost almost twenty pounds within two weeks; I did not want to eat nor could I sleep. I was lost. I wanted to curl up and die, to be with my Deedee. I built my life around her, we revolved around her. But when she passed, I lost my sense of purpose, like I had no one to take care of anymore. I became a stay-at-home mom so I could raise her, and give her my everything. We lived in San Antonio because of the great medical resources that assisted Dominique's growth. But when she passed, there was nothing left for us in San Antonio. So three months later we returned to Austin where Deedee was originally born.

At first I was angry at the world. I was mad that people acted like my daughter's death did not matter, no one paid attention to myself or my fiancé. But later on, after changing perspective and trying to appreciate that not everyone understands, I started to see what impact Dominique had in people's lives. She brought some kind of light to them, and it touched their heart.

It took some time, but I understood that Dominique's mission on Earth was done; that she had done what she came here to do. Sometimes I still struggle; she was gone way before she was supposed to.

I attended therapy and reached out to a couple of friends who had also lost children. I now understood the heart-felt pain they experience on a daily basis from not having their child with them. I wrote daily letters to Dominique in a notebook. I wrote about how much I missed her, and wished she were here with me.

I will be honest: I never saw myself as a survivor until the question asked how I survived the initial aftermath. I honestly thought that I wanted to die when Deedee passed. But I survived the tragedy of losing my only daughter. In doing so, I found a different sense of purpose: To help others and to share my experience, and try to teach people that life is precious.

*

MARY LEE CLAFLIN
Mary Lee's 2-month-old grandson Lane
died in 1998 from carbon monoxide poisoning

I was devastated. I cried all the time and finally got some much needed counseling. I needed to be able to live with the fact that I felt responsible for Lane's death. It took me over seventeen years to come to the answer I wanted for so long.

In the beginning, I would see my son Rob and his wife Charmayne and would start crying. I hurt for them as much as I did for myself. When my son was little, I could kiss away the hurt and he would go on with life. That was now impossible for me to do. I know we all grieve differently but I don't think Rob ever did fully. They ended up divorcing a couple of years later. My son said, "The baby lived, the baby died."

Since Rob could not stand to see me cry and I could not stop crying, we had to take a break from seeing each other. Lane died in January and I had already bought him his first Valentine's card but was never able to give it to him. I still have this card. I once read where they say the grandparents are the "forgotten grievers" and I believe this to be true most of the time.

*

ANNAH ELIZABETH
Annah Elizabeth's son Gavin Michael aspirated on his meconium during delivery in 1990 and died 26 minutes following his birth

My first experience with child loss came on an overcast, cold, dreary, yet otherwise truly magnetic day. I'd woken in the wee morning hours to what turned out to be real contractions, not those annoying Braxton Hicks pains. That labor progressed exactly as the books, doctors, and our Lamaze instructor had said it would. The room with its white walls and white linens, the bed with its stirrups, and the counter that held the doctor's plastic, examination gloves were all a part of the day's electric excitement.

One minute I was chatting with the nurse, only to watch her race from the room then return with what seemed like a posse of frantic people who informed my husband and I there was a problem with the baby and they were going to have to immediately perform surgery.

Dragging myself awake from that emergency cesarean section, I remember finally squeaking out these words: "Where's my baby?" "I'm sorry; he didn't make it," is the response forever burned into my brain.

Most of what I remember of the next week is blurred by a drug-induced haze. I had a few visitors, but only recently found out when I reconnected with an old friend that I had refused well-wishers in those earliest hours following Gavin's death. I remember reading condolence cards and weeping after I read the two Mother's Day cards friends sent. Two days following my son's birth

I should have been celebrating my new role as mommy. In joy's stead, one whisper filled every fiber of my being, one that rooted itself like an umbilical cord into my days and nights for a long time to come: What kind of mother has no child?

I survived the aftermath much like many of us do. I welcomed countless visitors that first week, then watched the well of company quickly dry up and the casseroles dry out. I cried buckets of tears and ate buckets of ice cream. I marveled at rainbows and hummingbirds and hated myself when I discovered I couldn't be happy for my sister who gave birth to my beautiful niece two weeks after my son died. I sat on the floor with Gavin's unused garments and rocked myself to sleep in our childless nursery. I went back to work, endured the panic-stricken looks from all those who didn't know or couldn't handle the fact that my son had died, and I welcomed the warm embraces from the few family and friends who could and would share in my sorrow.

I immediately chose to begin trying to have another baby. Seven years later I'd survived two more miscarriages, three complicated but successful pregnancies, and a six-week psychiatric stay for severe depression.

One of the questions that plagued me right from those earliest days in the hospital following Gavin's death was this: "How is it that some people can go on to live happy, healthy lives following tragedy while others succumb to despair, drugs, a life of void — or worse, suicide — and are forever held back from living their best lives?" Little by little I grew stronger and found numerous answers to that query. These are a few of the things I discovered.

We reduce grief to three words: "Loss and healing" or "grief and healing," when in essence there are three autonomous components. Loss equals the event. Grief equals our response to that loss event. Healing equals our recovery from the conflicts that comprise our grief. When we eliminate "loss" or "grief" we deny either the event or our sorrow.

Chinese philosopher, Lao Tzu once said, "The journey of a thousand miles begins with one step." Examining our daily language and understanding the autonomy between loss, grief, and healing are two of the first things we need to do on our road to recovery.

I realize our losses are often layered and I went on to identify five categories of loss: death, despair, disaster, disease and dysfunction. I also discovered that there are many nuances within each of those types of events. I discovered that each of us is born with everything we need to heal our big and small heartaches. I also noticed that, though the details look differently on each of us, we are all born with the same five traits: An academic ability to learn; we are born in a body and into a physical environment; we all have an ability to feel emotion and an ability to socialize in some form or another. Lastly, we are all born with a spirit.

Once I'd reconciled the last piece of my grief puzzle, I began assembling all of the grief event recovery tools I'd gathered on my journey. Helping others when their grief begins to soften has continued to help me through other life obstacles that have come my way.

*

NEISHA HART
Neisha's 6-month-old daughter
Brimley died in 2015 to SUID

At the time of this writing, is has been nine months since our daughter has passed, and time just seems to go on without slowing down. We kind of figured the first couple of days would be a whirlwind but it is almost like things are exactly the same, months passing us by when it seems like it should be days. The first month we leaned on each other. Family made sure we had what we needed and wanted so we didn't have to really think about anything. We both took an indefinite leave from work so we wouldn't have to see anyone or talk to anyone. We didn't know how to answer all the "I'm sorry," statements we were getting so we just avoided it. After the first month passed by, before we got the death certificate or autopsy results back, we wanted to blame each other. At the exact time the blaming was happening, it physically hurt. But it gave the other person a sense of relief to have someone to blame. That's what got us through the initial aftermath, and to be honest, I don't recommend anyone taking that path. The hurt and anger we felt toward each other was gut-wrenching.

*

BELINDA LUNA
Belinda's full-term baby Elijah
died in utero in 2012 from trisomy 18

Honestly I remember being in a very thick fog. Everything seemed so surreal and clouded to me. I was heavily medicated and just floating through my days. When I returned home everyone acted like it didn't happen. I went back into my shell so that I didn't make anyone uncomfortable.

*

MELISSA MEAD
Melissa's 13-month-old son
William died in 2014 from sepsis

I've handled the aftermath badly. Losing William has been an indescribable journey of survival. All I can hope for is to make it to the end of each day still breathing. There are times, and very often, that I don't want to be breathing, to be able to close my eyes and not wake up into this nightmare would be my dream. There is an enormous sense of not wanting to be here, but it isn't about a will or a wish to die, it is about being with William. I knew very shortly after William passed away that I couldn't do it on my own and was quickly under the care of the mental health team. My anxiety was uncontrollable; I could barely hold a glass of water without spilling its contents, and holding a pen wasn't a possibility. The adrenaline that constantly surged through my body kept me awake all night.

Then the flashbacks started. The moment I found William, the voice of the paramedic repeating the CPR instructions, 1 and 2 and 3 and 4, 1 and 2 and 3 and 4, rescue breath 1.....pause.... rescue breath 2..... and 1 and 2 and 3 and 4 and so on, the sounds of the paramedics flying up the stairs, the horror of watching invasive CPR on my baby, and those final words that shattered my life, "I'm sorry my love, but he's gone." These flashbacks are debilitating, leaves you unable to function and not part of society anymore.

Life for me is like I'm sitting in a side room watching what is going on through a window. The sounds are dulled, the people don't see me and I don't really take part. It has been ten months since William died, and I'm not living. I'm existing. The only aspect that has improved is that I can function a little better.

*

TAMARA NOVOTNY-KAUP
Tamara's 25-day-old daughter
Taylor Reanne died in 1995 of streptococcus

Taylor was twenty-five days-old when she passed away on a Sunday evening, January 8, 1995 at 6:06 p.m. I was frustrated, offended, embarrassed, angry, hurt, guilty and, of course, lost. I felt like I had all of this expectation and nothing to show for it and that I let my family down. I missed Taylor immediately. I felt frustrated with all of the unknowns. Why did this happen? What did I do wrong? Why won't anyone answer my questions? Why do I continually have more questions? Why is everyone upset with me for not having answers to *their* questions? Why do people keep asking me where my baby is? "No, I'm not fat. I just gave birth and no, she is not here anymore. Where is she? In heaven sir, she's in heaven." And then I was the one feeling awful for having to give such bad news all day, every day. Why do I feel bad for you feeling bad because you asked? I don't think there's any way to deliver such news, but I felt bad when others started the conversation. Would I have felt any less remorseful had I initiated the subject?

42

Again - why are there so many unanswered questions? My kids kept asking when we could bring Taylor home and each day I would tell them, "Soon, I hope." Well, after that it was even more difficult, as they called me a liar and then they'd cry. Here I am trying to deal with my loss, when it was our loss....I had no answers for them, I was lost. I turned to God to help me. I told the kids to pray, write down their questions and feelings and put them in a shoe box. I would read them while they were outside playing or when a grandparent came to take them out to keep them busy. I felt it "shelved" their feelings while giving me time to come up with a believable answer. It was a very difficult few months, but we all kept busy. I registered the kids for flag football, Boy Scouts and Girl Scouts. I'd like to think it helped us.

We did have another pregnancy between Taylor and our youngest, but it only lasted two months and I kept telling myself it was just too soon and it was meant to be. I don't know why we tell ourselves (and others) that it's meant to be. Who really knows that? I don't say that much anymore, but it helped back then as we made ourselves quite busy with extracurricular activities and it became an unattached memory in the back of our minds.

My husband chose to detach from Taylor after the first year of "firsts." He used to go with us to the cemetery, now he just says a prayer on her birthday. We don't talk about it. He doesn't want to, so I don't push. I have heard him mention her name in the past ten years or so, but it was more of in the form of a hypothetical, not a discussion. We gave up the idea that we would ever have another child, and started to accept that it was going to be the four of us now and continued forward. Then one day in 2001, I found out that I was pregnant. It was going to be different this time. And it was. I started to feel all of those feelings all over again, though. It was as if seven years ago was just last month. I cried a lot. I felt her kick. I was taken off of work so I had even more time to think about it. My only solution was listening to music and thank goodness for the internet too! I window shopped, I did buy some things. I did a lot of reading too. I started to feel guilty for being so happy that I'd made it farther along than my last pregnancy. So I started going back up to the cemetery to see Taylor. I took a snack, a baby magazine and blanket and sat at her gravesite. I went with and without the older two; we would talk to Taylor, and ask her questions. It started to make me feel better, so I went about once a week until I couldn't drive. Her older brother and sister became little experts on cutting the weeds and grass away from her marker, throwing away her old flowers and trimming her new ones. They'd sometimes fight to get the water and add new decorations. I never made them go with me, they often wanted to and I just hope it helped them as much as it helped me. I remember feeling the hole in my heart get a little smaller and the "weight" eased also. I may not talk about Taylor all of the time, but I do miss her all of the time.

I introduced Taylor's story to our youngest child when she discovered her photo album. I think she was about seven or eight years-old. We had our mini Q&A and she never seemed confused, only curious. She sometimes accompanies me when I go to see Taylor. She also now knows how to trim the weeds and get fresh water for her flowers. It makes it so much easier to talk about Taylor as if she's always around. She used to ask a lot of questions about Taylor. Now it's only once in a while. When I talk about her it seems to get easier. Our youngest has helped with our continued healing and she'll probably never know just how much.

*

SUSAN WILLIAMS
Susan's 2-month-old son
Tony died in 1987 from SIDS

I didn't handle the aftermath well. I'm sure adrenaline helped. I did what everyone told me to do. I was twenty-eight years-old, and had no idea what to do. I went to the funeral home, because that's what I was told to do. I couldn't talk, so my husband waited for me to nod yes or no to the questions asked by the funeral home director. We left the funeral home and went to the florist, because that's what they told me to do. When I got to the counter, I broke down and cried. Stu looked at me and I said: blue. He ordered a blue arrangement of carnations because that's what we could afford. On the day of the funeral, Stu's Aunt Sally (who had recently lost a son) asked me how I was doing. "Pretty s*****," was my reply. She said, "I was allowed." That was the first time I felt that my feelings were okay. I felt sh**y. I realized at that moment that her opinion mattered. She knew what it felt like to be me. She asked me if she could put a baby gold ring on Tony's finger that she had bought for him. That meant a lot to me. Aunt Sally knew what I was going through, and I was grateful for her gift.

Stu's sister and brother-in-law drove us to the wake and funeral which was on the same day. I remember sitting in the back seat just looking out the window thinking, "I am twenty-eight years-old, and I have to live with this for the rest of my life." I knew at that moment I would never be the same woman I was ever again. I just knew.

When Stu and I arrived at the funeral home, I really needed time alone with my son. I wasn't able to get it because everyone wanted to "save" Stu and I from the sorrow. Even though they meant well, they kept me from an intimate feeling that would have been a gift. We arrived in plenty of time to have some personal time with Tony, but unfortunately we didn't get it. Thank goodness, the funeral director gave us some time after everyone had left to say our final goodbye.

We took Zach to the funeral and wake. We had the only grandchildren at the time, and no one really knew what the right thing to do would be. I insisted on Zach being there. I know he was only two, but he lost his brother. I knew he would see his mom cry for the rest of her life. He needed to know why. I made the right call. In the Catholic religion they have a service but not a funeral Mass for the baby. They have an "angel" Mass about a month later. To this day, I'm not completely sure why they do this. Ironically, Tony was baptized two days before he died. I was going back to work, so I wanted to have him baptized so I could enjoy my family and friends seeing him being welcomed into the kingdom of Christ Jesus. Tony had a wake for approximately an hour, followed by a service that was given by our priest. After everyone had left the funeral home and were in their cars, Stu and I (holding Zach) had about ten minutes of the last "family time" we would ever have together for the rest of our lives.

As my brother-in-law drove us to the cemetery, I could not focus on anything except why I was twenty-eight years-old, and burying my son. Why? Why, God? Why is this happening to Stu and me? What did we do wrong?

March is cold. I got to the cemetery and it was freezing cold. They put my baby son in the freezing cold ground. Of course the priest said some comforting words, but I don't remember them. For crying out loud: they were putting my son in the freezing cold ground. My dad came over to stand by me, but no one came over to hug me or hold me. I was totally alone. They felt my pain. They could not comfort me, because they were hurting too much. I really needed to completely wrap myself in someone's arms and cry until I passed out. I totally get why no one stepped up to the plate, but I really wish someone would have had the courage to hold me.

My mom was totally my rock after the funeral. Shock helps for the first six weeks. I had to go back to work within a week, so I went. It was horrible to leave Zach at another babysitter after Tony died at a babysitter. I did not cope well.

*

CHAPTER THREE

THE FUNERAL

There is no foot too small that it cannot leave an imprint on this world. -UNKNOWN

For many the funeral represents the end while for others it marks the beginning of something eternal. Regardless of whether we mourn the absence of our child's physical body or celebrate the spirit that continues on, planning the funeral or memorial service presents emotionally-laden challenges shared by many.

*

DIANNA VAGIANOS ARMENTROUT
Dianna lost her newborn baby
Mary Rose in 2014 to trisomy 18

I planned a funeral while still pregnant. We had a coffin shipped to us from North Carolina. A couple whose son Joseph died at birth unexpectedly, made the baby coffin and sent it to our priest who was holding it until the funeral. That was a kindness – we didn't have the box in the house while waiting for Mary Rose's birth. We had a glitch in our plans though. The cemetery where we purchased the plot would only allow vaults, and the wooden casket was apparently illegal. If you could imagine an exhausted, tired, hungry woman who had just labored for over two days to hold her baby alive for less than an hour, a woman who was clutching her dead baby wrapped in a blanket with pink roses that said Mary Rose, finding out that she needed another casket. I was waiting for the pediatrician to come and pronounce my baby dead, so that I could dress her for burial. My midwife, husband and priest were on their cell phones talking loudly trying to sort this out. Our friend Annie has a friend who is a mortician, and Joe came by with an ugly gray plastic casket. My midwife and I cleaned Mary Rose with a damp cloth and rubbed baby lotion on her. My mother came in and helped me dress my daughter's cooling, stiffening body in her Victorian baptismal gown with pink roses. Her casket was on my bed. I put a tiny cross from my sister around her neck and gently laid her in the box. Father John tenderly carried Mary Rose down the stairs and out the door to take her body to church where people would read the psalms over her body through the night.

The next day the funeral was planned for two o'clock and we were late because of summer traffic. I was in a daze. We listened to the funeral service in the Eastern Orthodox tradition. Everyone kissed her goodbye and my husband would have been the last one to kiss her, but I bent down one more time and kissed her hand folded in the way of babies with trisomy 18. I carried her in my body, and I wanted to be the first and the last to kiss her. Father John put Mary Rose in his van and we drove to the cemetery.

There were more people there than I thought. My friend Yana came. My friend Paula was there. Joy came weeping because she had an ectopic pregnancy loss on August 8, 2008. She could not believe that Mary Rose died the same day, and she came to mourn her own baby at our funeral. I could not throw dirt at my baby. We left there before they lowered her into the ground. In our tradition we do memorial services at certain times after the death. We did a forty-day memorial service and then a one-year memorial service. I could not bring myself to do more, and I do not visit the cemetery much. I hate it there still.

With each miscarriage I took the membrane out of the toilet bowl, wrapped it in toilet paper and buried it under a statue of Our

Lady of Guadalupe outside. I did this in July. I did it again in October. I could not bear to name these two babies, as is recommended for healing. These two losses sit in the great shadow of their sister, Mary Rose. Recently I dreamt that I was birthing the two miscarried babies. My midwife tenderly took care of the membranes. I was told that the second baby, the one not born in October, had the name Politimi. This name means *precious* in Greek.

*

LINDA BATEMAN GOMEZ
Linda's 8-week-old son Chad
died in 1986 from SIDS

Surviving the funeral was difficult for me. I attended the meetings at the funeral home and I answered questions about flowers and write-ups when asked, but mostly I was just present, not really involved. Ernie did most of the actual planning. I didn't want to acknowledge the funeral because that made it real, yet I needed to be a part of it, as I knew it was the last thing I would be doing for my little Chad.

I also had major concerns about what would be best for my little girls, Tiffany and Krystle. Ernie's sister, Julie and our niece, Tisha, made sure that they were well taken care of which was so important to me. I was really worried about how all of this was affecting them. I was not sure about what was best as far as the services for the children, I knew they would need closure but what to do was a hard call. We took them briefly to the service and answered all of their questions as best we could for as young as they were.

It was really our immediate family that helped Ernie with the planning because it was all I could do to just be there. My Uncle Frankie was really organized and made sure that nothing was missed, there was so much paperwork and little details. It was all so calm and my dad being a funeral director was very helpful as well. It was as if they all just knew what to do and I was an observer.

My memories of those few days are scattered at best, with a few things really standing out in my mind. I remember picking daisies for the flowers which seemed so important and yet I have no idea why. Perhaps it was because it was one of the few decisions I actually made. Aside from the flowers, the music was really important to me. My Aunt Mary sang at the funeral and to this day I have no idea how she made it through the songs. Her voice was heaven sent and I remember feeling so at peace while she was singing, yet numb like I was in a daze.

I remember not having anything appropriate to wear for the funeral and my sister-in-law bought me a simple black dress, which I still have but have never worn again.

I never wanted Chad to be alone, so we purchased three spots in the mausoleum, one for Chad and one on each side of him for Ernie and myself as we were making the arrangements.

The actual funeral attendance was very large and I was in a fog at the services. I don't remember all of the details very clearly, but I do remember being in awe at the amount of people that traveled from all over the country to be there for him and us. I knew I needed to go through all of this, but I didn't even want to leave the house or get dressed, so to actually make it to the service felt like a big step. Luckily, I was blessed with the most wonderful family and friends in the world. The support that came was amazing and very much needed and appreciated.

My parents were divorced, but both my mother and father came together and were there for me, they even sat together at the funeral. Aside from Ernie and myself, I think my mother was most affected. I actually think her pain was doubled in some ways - for the loss of her grandchild and the hopeless pain she was witnessing in her own child, having no way to help stop it.

Oddly, I knew that Ernie was also hurting for me as well as himself. One of my strongest memories at the funeral was him hugging me and telling me he was sorry. While many other people said it that day, I knew from him it had deeper meaning. He worked so hard to save Chad that morning, and being a doctor I think made it even harder that he wasn't able to. He was hurting double, like my mother. Although the pain was overwhelming and nothing made me feel better, I knew I was surrounded by love.

For both Ernie and myself, it was having our family and friends at our side that helped us make it through the funeral. The funeral for me was my first step toward closure and the start of trying to figure out how life would move forward.

*

KARI BROWN
Kari's 2-year-old daughter Dominique (Deedee)
died in 2014 from obstructive sleep apnea

Brandon and I were in so much shock that it was difficult to determine the first step and how to go about planning a funeral, because we never thought we would have to plan a funeral for our child. We were not supposed to; our daughter was supposed to bury us. A good friend reached out to a few funeral homes and shared her findings with us. Brandon and I agreed on one funeral home. Brandon wanted to bury Dominique, but I wanted to cremate her because we loved to travel and we moved around a lot. I did not want to leave her behind. Eventually Brandon agreed to have Dominique cremated and, to this day, he is still grateful we made that decision. Wherever we travel, we take her urn with us as a physical reminder that she is always with us. Once we arrived at the funeral home, however, the assistant explained that it would be costly to order a coffin in her size and then cremate her. Brandon came up with the idea of using Dominique's crib instead of a coffin, and then she would be cremated without additional cost. It was difficult picking out an urn, because we were still in a state of shock and feeling so unreal that this was happening. Family members helped set up the crib along with Dominique's body surrounded by her favorite toys.

During the wake, I felt somewhat relieved that she was laid to rest in her crib and not in a coffin, because she looked like she was sleeping. During the wake we held her hand and I started to feel warmth in her hand, like she was coming back to me. I prayed and prayed she would just wake up. But that didn't happen; the heat from my hand warmed up hers. I begged and begged for her to wake up, to come back to us. But that didn't happen.

We wrote the eulogy, however as I read it today, I am a little dissatisfied. It seemed unorganized and a bit rushed. We know what Dominique means to us, what she means to other people, and how much love she brought into our lives. The day she was scheduled to be cremated, it was an ugly day; it was gloomy and cloudy. When Brandon and I walked to the front of the building where cremations took place, a ray of sunlight shone on my feet and then faded away. I cried, knowing it was a sign: Dominique was telling us that it was okay. She was placed in a small pink urn with three white doves etched in it. It's a simple but beautiful place for her remains to be in.

*

MARY LEE CLAFLIN
Mary Lee's 2-month-old grandson Lane
died in 1998 from carbon monoxide poisoning

My daughter and I went along with my son Rob and his wife Charmayne to arrange the service. I knew this funeral home well, as I worked at the church and they did many funerals with us. They have a standard casket for babies that they supply for the burial. It is not pretty by any means. When Charmayne saw it she started crying. She said she could not bury her baby in that. We talked with the funeral director and he let her pick out a maple casket and did not charge us for it. Their kindness and generosity helped to make this experience a little more bearable. The church had been given some cemetery plots so we bought one to use for Lane. Since Rob and Charmayne did not belong to a church, we had the service at the church I worked at and was a member of.

*

ANNAH ELIZABETH
Annah Elizabeth's son Gavin Michael aspirated on his meconium
during delivery in 1990 and died 26 minutes following his birth

I spent nearly a week in the hospital following the emergency cesarean section that brought my son into this world. Those days are really a blur for me…a combination of the shock and the drugs used to help keep me as calm as possible so I wouldn't do damage to my incision.

As such, my husband made most of the funeral arrangements like talking with the funeral home, choosing a casket, listening to the steps we needed to take, making preparations for a burial plot, gathering information that he could bring back to me at the hospital. Together we chose the headstone.

One of the documents someone gave us in the first few days after Gavin died suggested that we write farewell letters to our child. So we did. Warren and I also wrote personal letters to our boy. Always a writer at heart, I also penned a poem that the minister included in the burial service, along with my goodbye letter that was written more as a we'll-see-you-later-send-off-letter than a goodbye.

The only reason I recollect any of this is because I made photocopies of everything and placed them in the box with the few mementoes the hospital had collected for me and Warren…baby's first blanket…Baby Boy Fleming's bassinet card…his little knitted cap and the paper tape measure they used to record his birth statistics…articles that serve as living testimony of our experiences, both good and bad…

We held the service in a small chapel attached to our church. Warren and I arrived early to spend our last minutes with our boy before his burial, and then invited anyone who wanted to pay their respects an opportunity to do so. We placed a few photos, toys, and a baby book in his casket before taking our places in the pews. The skies wept hard as we arrived at the cemetery, making the trek up the hillside difficult for me, so we sat in our car and watched our son's body being lowered into the ground. I remember thinking how befitting the rain was in light of the tears shed that day.

*

NEISHA HART
Neisha's 6-month-old daughter
Brimley died in 2015 to SUID

For the initial funeral planning session it was Brad and I, my parents, and Brad's parents. My one wish was to have Brimley's funeral at the local funeral home in my hometown. I knew my mind could rest for just a couple of days knowing Brimley was in good hands before I saw her again.

My family had two cemetery plots already claimed for my mother and my father. The two had gone through a divorce many years before, so there was one open plot. There was no doubt in my mind I wanted Brimley buried there. In future years to come, I know there would be no better place than having her placed between my grandmother and my mother.

Being a twenty-three-year-old, I had no idea what went on when planning a funeral, and never thought I would have to do it for my child. The amount of things we had to choose between, from which color casket, what clothing to put her in, diaper or no diaper, shoes and socks or neither. Some of the things were everyday no-brainers when I was caring for my child, but making the choice for the very last time, knowing I could never change that choice was overwhelming to say the least. Between Brad and me, I kind of took charge in the planning and decision making because that is who I am. I need to feel in control all the time.

*

BELINDA LUNA
Belinda's full-term baby Elijah
died in utero in 2012 from trisomy 18

We were unable to have a service for Elijah. Something I will have to live with the rest of my life.

*

MELISSA MEAD
Melissa's 13-month-old son
William died in 2014 from sepsis

I planned the funeral along with William's father, Paul. We decided that we would like to have William cremated, although we didn't want that either. But the thought of burying William in the ground and leaving him there, cold and alone was terrifying. I knew I wouldn't leave his side. It felt only right for us to bring him home. So we did.

I visited William every day in the Chapel of Rest. I held him every time, I cuddled him, I talked to him, I cried on him and I showed him my love. After all, he was still my baby, and my baby needed me.

During the funeral I read two poems and a letter to William, and we recorded the service so that if I wanted to, I could watch it. It was a good job and I recorded it as if there was no one in that room other than me and my boy. Watching those curtains close at William's funeral, knowing that I would never see him again destroyed me.

William's ashes are now safely in a beautiful silver heart, inside of a lovely teddy bear that I cuddle every night. Planning William's funeral wasn't easy, in fact it is the most conflicting thing ever. Something you absolutely do not want to do, but something you know you have to get right, and something that is special.

*

SUSAN WILLIAMS
Susan's 2-month-old son
Tony died in 1987 from SIDS

The funeral director was amazing. She included her husband in everything she did with the business. He founded the business, but had recently had a major stroke. He was limited in his speech, but she included him in all the "director" duties. She taught me the gift of dignity. I was totally in shock that day, but I remember that act of love.

I could not make any decisions, and she steered Stu and I in the right direction. I thought she was amazing with two young parents who just lost their baby boy. I wrote this wonderful woman a letter years after the death of our son, telling her how much she taught me that day. Her dear husband passed a couple of years after our son. He must have been a wonderful man.

*

CHAPTER FOUR

THE TRANSITION

The bereaved need more than just the space to grieve the loss. They also need the space to grieve the transition. - LYNDA CHELDELIN FELL

As we begin the transition of facing life without our child, some find comfort by immediately returning to a familiar routine, while others find solitude a safe haven. Sometimes our own circumstances don't allow choices to ponder, and we simply follow where the path leads. But the one commonality we're all faced with is the starting point that marks the transition from our old life to the new.

*

DIANNA VAGIANOS ARMENTROUT
Dianna lost her newborn baby
Mary Rose in 2014 to trisomy 18

My husband took one week off and then threw himself back into his work. He was not able to support me much during those postpartum months. (Thankfully, I have an awesome therapist.) I realize now that he could not cope with this loss any better than he did. It took a long time for him to be able to talk about Mary Rose. He was not dealing with the grief as I was during the pregnancy. He had work and his exercise. His routine was very important to his moving on.

He was able to distract himself during the pregnancy, while I carried our daughter who would die in my own body. It took months for my husband and I to be on the same page about our daughter's life and death. He could not grieve openly as I did, and he didn't have a postpartum body. As he grieved privately and I stepped out of the fog of shock slowly we were able to be together peacefully as a couple, but it took time. I needed to cocoon myself away from the world. I did go to church and to one moms' group, but everything was difficult for me. I don't think I will ever transition back into the life I had before I held life and death in my arms for one life-changing moment.

*

LINDA BATEMAN GOMEZ
Linda's 8-week-old son Chad
died in 1986 from SIDS

The year that followed was the longest year of my life, and probably for friends and family as well, especially my husband. The first three months were the hardest and very robotic, I just did what I had to do. The support of my husband was incredible though. He allowed me to do what I needed to get through.

Because I was a stay-at-home mom, I didn't do anything except stay inside and spend every second with my little girls. The only other place I would go was the cemetery as I found comfort there.

My husband handled his grief totally different. It was hard for me to understand at the time, though I do now of course. Everyone handles it differently and there is no right or wrong. Some people need to talk or visit the gravesite, while others find that too painful to do. Some want to sit and cry, others need to stay busy and not think about it. It is all okay, and you need to do whatever is necessary for you personally to get through it. In my case, my husband and I were total opposites. He went back to work and didn't want to talk about it. I had no outside work to go to and all I wanted to do was talk about Chad. I was looking for answers and not finding them. We were both surrounded by family and friends, and although sometimes they tried to help in ways that didn't, we knew we had a lot of love and support and that really helped.

While struggling and grasping for answers, I knew in my heart I had to look toward the future. I had to find a way to transition back into being a mother who now only had two children, not three. In my need for comfort and to understand how to move forward, I found myself reading anything I could for answers. I wanted to better understand SIDS and the grieving process. I needed to know how to help my girls understand. I also wrote songs and poems about Chad because I found comfort in that. I wanted to make sure I kept Chad's memory alive and one way I could was with photos. My Uncle Frankie had my favorite picture blown up and gave one to all the family members, it remains on my dresser today. In order to make the transition back into everyday life, I needed assurance that at no point Chad's memory would be left behind. For me, I think as a stay-at-home mom, because I had no outside job and my entire life and reason for living revolved around my children, it took me the better part of the year to really feel like I had fully adjusted. While it wasn't as fast for me as it was for my husband, I made it. It just took me a little more time. Slow and steady, at my own pace and my own way, I finally made it.

*

MARY LEE CLAFLIN
Mary Lee's 2-month-old grandson Lane
died in 1998 from carbon monoxide poisoning

The funeral was on a Saturday and I returned to work the following Monday. I was only allowed three days for in-town services, and had already missed four days. People would come into my office and offer their sympathy and the tears would flood my eyes. It was difficult being around people those first few weeks. I did feel their love and support for my loss. I received many sympathy cards. Even more special were the people who wrote notes, telling me of their grandbaby's death and what the world would be like for me in years to come, how I would be able to see another baby without crying. They said that I would hold a baby again and be able to trust that life would not always be like this, that the hurt would subside and God would be there for me always.

*

ANNAH ELIZABETH
Annah Elizabeth's son Gavin Michael aspirated on his meconium during delivery in 1990 and died 26 minutes following his birth

Though the details look differently on the various types of child loss, I do believe that the death of a child occurs whether that child is eight weeks gestation, a full-term baby or an eight-year-old when he or she expires. Having experienced the death of a living child as well as two miscarriages, my experiences vary. I eased back into work following my son's death and went back full time when the doctor released me eight weeks after the emergency cesarean section. If memory serves me right, I returned to work within a day or two following both miscarriages.

During my grief periods that followed the death of my son and both miscarriages, I was fortunate to be working for a small family-owned business. The family offered me a great deal of support, comfort, and understanding. For me, work helped keep my mind focused on other things besides my loss. I didn't want to sit at home and wallow in self-pity, so having tasks to accomplish during the day helped to manage the time I spent grieving and provided me a sense of success.

I felt needed, valued, appreciated, competent, and trusted at work, emotions that offset those feelings of inferiority and shame that came with my grief. Don't get me wrong, I'm sure I had sad spells during the day — when a particular song came on, a pregnant woman came into the office, or a customer came in with a baby in hand, but in the bigger picture, my visible grief came outside of office hours, so to speak. For me, especially in the aftermath of my son's death, being able to return to work and have something to focus on helped me through my initial suffering.

Because of their empathy and understanding, my employers allowed me to perform a few simple paperwork tasks at home, even before I was released to go back to work after the emergency surgery that brought my eldest child into this world. This allowed me the freedom to grieve when I needed to while still affording me opportunity to feel a sense of accomplishment. The interaction with others also helped stave off that overwhelming sense of isolation and aloneness that accompanies significant sorrow. I am eternally grateful for those transition and therapeutic pieces that I was afforded in my employment.

*

RENEE FORD-ROMERO
Renee's son Diego was stillborn due
to an undiagnosed cardiac fibroma in 2014

I've been in the same Department of Defense building with the same crew for seven years. Our work is stressful and intense and out of that environment, pretty strong bonds with one another are formed. Returning to work after the two losses where I took substantial leave were two very different experiences. While home recovering after my second trimester loss I got flowers, a few visits, tons of phone calls and texts. I felt supported. During the recovery from Diego's birth, I got one text message from an unlikely source, a gentleman probably more concerned with fueling the rumor mill than sincerely checking on me. Unbeknownst to me, someone in another department started a rumor that I had quit, and a supervisor in that same area said that I had requested not to be contacted. All this was going on without my knowledge for six weeks, so naturally I was hurt and angry! I thought how could these people, my friends, these coworkers I spent nine hours a day with for seven years be so cold? My boss cleared it up and the team of folks I work closest with quickly apologized and were very supportive.

I leaned on my church family. I look back at it now and I see how God used something painful to free me from my paid job and prepare me for my volunteer work. He removed some of the damaging rumor-starting, chaos-loving people from my life. It was painful at the time but I'm ultimately so grateful. I'm so much better at boundaries. I no longer feel obligated to work outside my schedule and my stress level is so much lower! I know it was a rumor, a misunderstanding, but a blessing in disguise nonetheless.

For the other hundred or so people outside of my immediate area, their reaction upon my return was shock because they thought I had quit. After I explained that I hadn't quit, that it was a false rumor, the natural reaction was a big fat congratulations and an inquiry as to how my son was doing. So for several months, sometimes multiple times a day, I had to "break the news" to random people that my son had passed away. Talk about awkward hallway conversation. I didn't mind so much in the restroom, at least I could hide in the stall and cry in private. It got to the point where I came in, headed straight to my desk and stayed out of public areas as much as possible. I still do.

Another blessing in disguise is that I'm way more productive now. For my little girl, there was no silver lining needed. We've been very careful not to expect her emotional maturity to match ours, but she amazes me daily. She is so resilient. She did a year of bereavement group therapy with other children her age. After we lost our son, she was such a trooper. She stuck it out and finished up the last two weeks of the school year.

After that last miscarriage though, at the end of summer, we took a trip to the coast to rest and spend some quality time together. God blessed us with a beautifully upgraded condo, discounts on everything, no crowds; He absolutely paved the way for a relaxing few days. Our daughter missed the first couple days of the next school year, I take full responsibility but I'm not apologizing. We needed a break and I misread the dates that school was to start. She's a straight A student, wins every contest, earns awards, sings like a bird, reads three grades higher than her classmates, so a few days off didn't hurt one bit.

When I took her to school for her first day, a few days late, the school administration would not excuse her absence. I am usually very calm, collected, and professional; I don't make scenes. But that little girl behind the desk who looked like she barely graduated school herself picked the wrong day and the wrong woman to berate about a child missing the first days of school to play at the beach. My response was probably sparked by a combination of rage and hormones, and (God forgive me) I'm pretty sure the entire school heard. That day my daughter witnessed what a mama lion looks like when you mess with her cub.

*

NEISHA HART
Neisha's 6-month-old daughter
Brimley died in 2015 to SUID

Brad and I both decided to take a minimum of two weeks off work to avoid unwanted situations and be able to get through the day without breaking down. After the two weeks passed, I went back to Child Protective Services where I was doing my internship for my final semester of college. Just being there made me so anxious and overwhelmed, I decided to pause my internship and withdraw from my classes for the semester. I am glad I did because now that I have returned, I don't have any of those negative feelings toward being in the office like I used to. Brad tried to go back to work but it was just too emotional for him. His daily routine was to get Brimley up in the morning, feed her, change her, and get her dressed for the day. On his way to work, they would have their daily jam session in the truck before he would drop her off at daycare. I can't even begin to imagine what he went through every day, going through the same routine without his little girl. After a little bit, the guilt began to set in on Brad and affect his sleeping schedule. Brad was awake that whole night that Brimley passed away and he feels guilty that he couldn't stop it. But what he has to realize is there was nothing we could have done to stop it. It happens to parents who are in the same room as their child, and the baby never makes a sound, just as Brimley didn't.

Nine months later we are both still struggling, but we are improving more and more each day. I am working full time at a local hotel and finishing up my internship hours at Child Protective Services. Brad is still searching for that one special job he loves to do and looks forward to being at every day. Hopefully it will come soon and we can get our lives back on, well a different track, and focus on the goals we set for ourselves.

*

BELINDA LUNA
Belinda's full-term baby Elijah
died in utero in 2012 from trisomy 18

I still have not returned to work almost three years later!!! I'm frightened of being back out there in the world.

*

MELISSA MEAD
Melissa's 13-month-old son
William died in 2014 from sepsis

Paul, William's father, returned to work after several months, whereas I took a lot longer, possibly six months. I am lucky that I have an amazing boss, who happens to be William's godfather. I was able to just ease myself back in at my own pace. Some days it was too much, and I went home or stared at the wall. It is always better to sit at work and stare at the wall than sit at home on my own staring at the wall. Being at work does give me a focus, but it is extremely hard to concentrate and I forget things, most things in fact. I don't have any motivation or drive anymore. I don't put pressure on myself to be "better" tomorrow than I am today, because as we have found out, tomorrow is never promised. I will deal with tomorrow when it comes around.

*

SUSAN WILLIAMS
Susan's 2-month-old son
Tony died in 1987 from SIDS

The worst and best thing I ever did in my life was go back to work. At the time, I wanted someone to tell me that I could stay home with Zach. Wasn't that the answer? I couldn't be expected to bring Zach to another sitter. How could he or I cope with that? But that's exactly what happened. I can't blame it on anything except finances. Stu and I built a house on a beautiful piece of land two years before Tony was born. It did not even have air conditioning yet, but it was set up for it. When we mortgaged the home, both Stu and I had steady full-time jobs. After five years of teaching music, my school corporation reduced all art, P.E., and music teachers. I was suddenly unemployed. I received unemployment checks until I found a part-time position forty-five minutes away from home. I felt it was a blessing at the time. I didn't get paid well, but I got to spend more time with Zach. Plus, I was expecting a new baby soon.

My new job was set up like this: I taught grades one through five twice a week and grades nine through twelve band every day. I also taught a high school girls chorus that met every day. One of the girls was pregnant when I came back after Tony had died. I really had a hard time with that. I continued to question God on this matter. Why was he so unfair? Why could an unwed mother be in front of me every day to remind me that I was being punished? That is how I felt at the time. Later, I would learn that she deserved to bring a child into the world just as much as I did. Years down the road, this girl stopped me and introduced me to her husband and two children. She married the father of that child, and had another child as well. They were a very happy family.

The teachers, staff, and parents were amazing to me when I came back. Hugs and comfort were given freely. My principal was amazing. I had a couple of hard days, and I was able to leave without feeling guilty. I was blessed with wonderful loving people who helped me get through the next three months.

After three months, I Interviewed for a higher paying job that was closer to home. I got the job, but will always be grateful for the love this staff provided for me. A year after I left this wonderful staff, the principal of that school and his wife lost their son to a virus. At the time, their son was in the military. They flew him back to Indiana to get better medical help, but he died within a short amount of time. This principal was the same one that made sure his staff encouraged me to just do my best. If I was having a bad day, they picked me off the ground and helped me through the day. Now, the tables were turned over. I was still raw in my grief, but I was able to go to their son's funeral and follow up with support. I'm not sure how it all happened, other than we shared the same nightmare. Stu and I still love to visit them even though they live about fifty minutes away. They are family to us.

The next year and the years following, I preferred to concentrate on my students and not bring my story to work. I would tell my new coworkers that I only had one son, so I didn't wreck their day. I felt so guilty doing this. When I connected closely with someone, I told them about Tony. I guess you had to be Tony-worthy for me to allow you into my life. It was hard to love anyone new. I loved my son so much, and he was taken away from me. I just didn't have the courage to start new relationships. But, somehow I did. I was blessed with many people in the first two sorrowful years who helped me be the best teacher I could be even though I was going through the most painful time of my life.

I never thought about how totally blessed I was because these special people were put on my life at that particular time until I put these words down for this article. Thank you for this blessing! May God bless these special people!

*

CHAPTER FIVE

THE QUESTION

Grievers use a very simple calendar. Before and after. - LYNDA CHELDELIN FELL

One day we have a baby. The next, our precious child is no longer living. How do we explain to others something we can't wrap our brains around? And how do we answer the question that appears simple to everyone but us: How many children do you have?

*

DIANNA VAGIANOS ARMENTROUT
Dianna lost her newborn baby
Mary Rose in 2014 to trisomy 18

People don't want to hear about Mary Rose or my miscarriages. I always mention Mary Rose when asked how many children I have. Oh, the look of horror on people's faces! How dare I mention a dead baby? I do speak of my miscarriages, but they come up less often, and also make people uncomfortable. I think that for people who think that I should just have another child to make up for the loss of Mary Rose, the miscarriages leave them speechless. How could one person face so much loss? People don't know what to say or do as they grow their own families and continue on with their lives.

*

LINDA BATEMAN GOMEZ
Linda's 8-week-old son Chad
died in 1986 from SIDS

When people ask me how many children I have, my answer varies depending on the situation and my mood at the time. The majority of the time I answer that I have six children, five living. When I answer this way it is often met with an awkward response. Sometimes people say, "I'm sorry." Other times they ask what happened. Sometimes they seem uncomfortable because they aren't sure what to say, which of course is never my intention.

If I decide, for whatever reason at the time, that I don't want to answer questions about Chad's death, I simply say five. It depends much on why they are asking. I have found over time that if they happen to probe deeper and ask what my children do, school or workwise, or how old they are, I know it will get awkward. When there are only five responses to give, it naturally opens the door to more questions about the sixth child, which I may or may not want to answer. It really just depends on who is asking and how I am feeling at the time. Sometimes I don't mind answering questions and other times I don't want to go down that path. While I never like to have anyone feel uncomfortable, some days I just need to acknowledge that I have "six children, five living" so that is most often my answer. I must admit though that when I answer five, I always feel a little guilty. I don't ever want to leave Chad out, but of course I know that I am not, it's simply the typical mother's guilt.

*

KARI BROWN
Kari's 2-year-old daughter Dominique (Deedee)
died in 2014 from obstructive sleep apnea

I've always had difficulty answering the question about how many children I have. At this time I have my only daughter, Dominique, who's not here with me. However, the answer to the question varies based on who is asking, and where I am at the moment. Sometimes I talk about Dominique as if she were still alive. It also depends on the "vibe" I'm feeling from the person who is asking the question. If I feel confident and comfortable enough to explain about my daughter, I will. If I am having one of those hard days, I may say nothing at all. It also depends on my mindset when I wake up in the morning; I may bravely battle the emotions boiling up in me, or I may let my guard down and cry when asked. But I never fail to hesitate at answering such questions. No matter how prepared I may be, or how much I practice the answer in my mind, I always hesitate. I feel guilty if I don't honestly explain the situation. My daughter passed a year and a half ago. And I still hesitate at the same question.

*

MARY LEE CLAFLIN
Mary Lee's 2-month-old grandson Lane
died in 1998 from carbon monoxide poisoning

I answer I have eleven grandchildren. One is living in Heaven and the others here on earth. I will always consider Lane as one of my grandchildren because he is. In the beginning I would be sad to tell people he had died. Now when I think about him, I can smile. I am so thankful of the time we had with him. I just wish it could have been longer.

*

ANNAH ELIZABETH
Annah Elizabeth's son Gavin Michael aspirated on his meconium
during delivery in 1990 and died 26 minutes following his birth

This is a question that has many answers, each dependent on the situation. Though I'm not quick to reveal that I have experienced child loss in the forms of miscarriage and infant death, I don't withhold the information, either. In the earlier years I would most often respond that I had three children, sometimes saying, "I have three living children." If I was in a passing conversation, one that I expected to pass quickly, I would speak the former. If, however, I were in a casual conversation or getting to know someone new, I would give the latter reply.

In the past ten years, since I began my work on healing grief, I have begun more often than not to reply that I have four children. If the conversation turns to, "What do they do?" I start off with my youngest child, who just graduated high school, and then work my way up. When I get to the eldest, I usually say something like, "My eldest died shortly after he was born and lives with us in spirit." I remember once, when I met someone with whom I was joking about parenting hardships and someone I immediately identified to have a great sense of humor, I replied, "My eldest is wreaking havoc in heaven." More often than not, the conversation will then turn to the subject of miscarriage and other forms of fertility topics. I am constantly amazed by how often the conversation comes up and I am equally inspired and pleasantly surprised by the number of people who will open up and share their experiences with me once I've opened up the discussion.

*

RENEE FORD-ROMERO
Renee's son Diego was stillborn due to
an undiagnosed cardiac fibroma in 2014

You can't exactly hide the fact that where there had been a big old belly, there's now just empty space. With the earlier losses, I was ashamed and even afraid to tell my friends and family I was pregnant yet again, but God started putting women in my path with this same hurt (like every day) and I do not believe in coincidence. I know there's a reason but I'm fleshy and selfish and semi-private and a major smart aleck! It's uncomfortable and personal to talk about this kind of loss with other women, but I submitted to the fact that there's a reason these woman now flock to me. He keeps putting 2 Corinthians 1:3 and 4 in front of me.

It says, *"Praise be to the God and Father of our Lord Jesus Christ, the Father of compassion and the God of all comfort, 4 who comforts us in all our troubles, so that we can comfort those in any trouble with the comfort we ourselves receive from God."*

God's supernatural comfort came to me in the form of an army of Christian sisters who loved me, fed my family, cleaned my house, and even comforted my daughter when I was being strangled by grief. They are the perfect example of what I need to be to these women who God is putting in my path so often now. Even non-Christians know the story of Job and the kind of "friends" he had. For three verses though, he has really good friends. They traveled to be with him, they tore their robes and they mourned with him in silence for seven days. That's a HUGE deal! BUT then they opened their mouths. And when they did, out comes the same kind of bologna that exists in conversations with myself sometimes, "God's not answering your prayers because of your past, this is punishment for sin, you don't deserve a baby."

I was at a women's bible study not long after I lost my son and as I sat there surrounded by so many women, that self-conversation changed. Yes, these women are wounded, but they're warriors! Unlike Job's friends, these spiritual mothers and sisters fiercely rebuke the enemy and speak restoration and healing over me and my family. These girls make me laugh. I can't stay sad when I've got these awesome women in my life. They are a living breathing testament to God's love for me and His faithfulness to those who are faithful to Him and I am so grateful to Him.

*

NEISHA HART
Neisha's 6-month-old daughter
Brimley died in 2015 to SUID

I would go crazy inside if I couldn't talk about my daughter, our family, or our story. I work at a hotel in my hometown and we often have guests who are in town for funerals. I am able to connect with my guests on a deeper level once I open up and let them know that I truly know what they are going through. My other staff tell me they wish they would get guests to open up like I can, but we have something in common I would never wish upon anyone.

I often tell my story for others to learn from my loss. At times my emotions can creep up and overwhelm me, but I seem more comfortable now with what happened. I'm able to talk about it, and I seem to be able to control my emotions a lot better now.

I do have conversations with those who I never felt the need to hold back my emotions, or need to see me at my worst, to realize what I am really feeling. People often say to me that I am very strong and deal with the emotions well. Most of the time they are right. The other times, I just don't let anyone see me at my worst. Brad and I started a YouTube series, *Living With Child Loss*, just so our friends and family can get a peek inside our current lives without being too invasive, as they would call it.

*

BELINDA LUNA
Belinda's full-term baby Elijah
died in utero in 2012 from trisomy 18

I have four children, three here on earth and one in heaven.

*

MELISSA MEAD
Melissa's 13-month-old son
William died in 2014 from sepsis

When someone asks me how many children I have, I always answer one. If they go on to ask further questions, I always answer truthfully. Is it a boy or a girl? I have a little boy. Most questions can be answered without prompting a sharp inward breath. If they ask how old he is, I answer, "William is forever one," and then go on to say that he passed away.

I know that some people choose to not go further or not include their angel child in the conversation but for me that is not something I can do. Equally, if anyone feels awkward, it is never me. Some people don't know what to say, others offer standard sentiments, others apologize profusely. Nothing anyone can say can make the situation worse, people can't possibly "remind" me that my son has passed away. I live with it through every moment of each day. I see it as an opportunity to share William with another person, to be able to describe to them how perfect William was, and to be able to show them a photo. When I hear the words, "He's so beautiful," it fills me with so much pride.

*

SUSAN WILLIAMS
Susan's 2-month-old son
Tony died in 1987 from SIDS

In the first raw years, that question was gut-wrenching. I attended a support group, The Compassionate Friends, early in my grief. They helped me decide for myself how to answer this question. It's totally personal to the bereaved parent how they answer it. Most of the time, it's a matter of thinking about the person who asked the question.

I always asked myself "Do I really want to ruin their day?" If I know this person is going to be someone that I care about, and will benefit from knowing about my son Tony, then I put my big girl panties on and pray they are worthy of sharing in the love I have for my son.

*

Just as it is impossible to explain childbirth
to a woman who has never given birth,
it is impossible to explain child loss
to a person who has never lost a child.
LYNDA CHELDELIN FELL

*

CHAPTER SIX

THE DATES

If there ever comes a day when we can't be together,
put me in your heart, I'll stay there forever.
-A. A. MILNE, WINNIE THE POOH

Our expectations and memories of balloons and cakes and presents are as regular as the rising sun. When our child passes, however, how do we celebrate the life that is no more? And how do we acknowledge the painful date that marks their death?

*

DIANNA VAGIANOS ARMENTROUT
Dianna lost her newborn baby
Mary Rose in 2014 to trisomy 18

I had a few friends over on the first anniversary of Mary Rose's birth and death. It is the same date. August 8, 2014. It was a potluck and we talked and hung out. I didn't plan any activity or sing "Happy Birthday." I just wanted people around me to remember her life. People who had witnessed Mary Rose's existence – people who knew that she was *real*. I don't know how we will acknowledge this going forward. It is her birthday still, as Heidi Faith says on her website *Still*birthday. We will continue to do memorials for her on the one-year anniversary at church.

I think that this year I might want a quiet day to remember. I don't know if I will acknowledge the miscarriages. It feels like too much loss to bear and remember.

July. August. October. It's a lot to process.

*

LINDA BATEMAN GOMEZ
Linda's 8-week-old son Chad
died in 1986 from SIDS

Those are both still very hard days for me, even after all of these years. What's funny is that it's the two weeks leading up to them that seems harder for me than the actual days. I become very irritable; it's almost like subconsciously I'm thinking about them before I even realize it's that close. There is no question to the rest of the family that something is up. Once the day comes and goes, both the death and birthday, it's like closure and proof yet again that I can make it through.

What we do on those days has changed over the years. For about the first ten years after Chad died, we always released balloons and took flowers to the cemetery with the whole family. Now, with the other children all grown, it is rare that we all make it out at the same time, so we usually go in smaller groups. My husband and myself take the flowers, visit at his site, and say a prayer with whatever siblings can join us.

As of this writing, it has been twenty-nine years and those days are still hard. Not only because I miss him, but because I'm sad for all the things he missed out on. I still cry.

*
KARI BROWN
Kari's 2-year-old daughter Dominique (Deedee)
died in 2014 from obstructive sleep apnea

The very first birthday Dominique was not here was heart-wrenching. I was overwhelmed and torn that she was not here for her third birthday. My mother-in-law purchased a ranch and wanted to bless it on Dominique's birthday. So we decorated the ranch in purple and white balloons, and put together a special cake with the number three on it. Later that evening, we took turns speaking about Dominique and the impact she had on each of us. We then released a bundle of balloons and watched as they floated away in the sunset; I wished I could have floated away to her too.

For her first "angelversary," my fiancé and I had mixed emotions about what we should do, or how we should celebrate it. We ended up doing a simple photoshoot with bluebonnets, a canvas print of Dominique, and her urn along with her favorite boots. I've always wanted to take pictures of Dominique in bluebonnets because it is the state flower of Texas, but I never got the opportunity. We felt that honoring her in a field of bluebonnets was a special way to remember her. I think our rituals will be different every year, depending on how we feel when the time comes around.

*
MARY LEE CLAFLIN
Mary Lee's 2-month-old grandson Lane
died in 1998 from carbon monoxide poisoning

I would always go to the cemetery on Lane's birthday and the day he died. Sometimes when I got there, I would see that his mother or his other grandmother had been there with flowers. Lane's mother Charmayne never misses going to the cemetery for all occasions. I would clean off any dirt on his marker and then would remember the first two months of his life starting with his birth. I remember that I was not ready to be a grandmother and told him what joy he brought into my life. I had gone through a terrible divorce and for the first time in many years he gave me hope for the future and a reason to be glad to be alive.

*

ANNAH ELIZABETH
Annah Elizabeth's son Gavin Michael aspirated on his meconium during delivery in 1990 and died 26 minutes following his birth

Gavin died twenty-six minutes following his birth, so both of these events fall on the same day. We always buy a few balloons and some special spring decoration, since his special day falls on the heels of winter's end. We pull unwanted weeds from around his grave marker, we pad the empty space with pine needles, and set out the gifts we brought. Since he was born so close to Mother's Day, I decided to have each of my other children baptized on Mother's Day. It was a way for me to celebrate the life of each new life while honoring the memory of another.

On Gavin's twenty-first birthday we went to a special restaurant we'd never visited before and I had a chocolate raspberry martini in his honor. I commissioned a painting in honor of Gavin's twenty-fifth birthday; a creative work that captured one of our conversations we had during an earlier birthday visit to Gavin's grave.

One of my most special traditions, though, is how we form a circle around his stone. Hands held, we wonder aloud about things Gavin might be doing in heaven, what toys he would have been playing with or, when he became of driving age, what kind of car he'd be driving. We take turns sending Gavin a special message. I've always believed that Gavin's spirit is with us wherever we are, so visiting the cemetery is more of a formality for us, but it is the tradition that my three living children have always known and it is one they've always remembered.

*

NEISHA HART
Neisha's 6-month-old daughter
Brimley died in 2015 to SUID

June 25th of each year will always be my baby's birthday. For every year to come. Just this past year, what would have been her first birthday, we told her happy birthday and took flowers and balloons to the cemetery. I always want that date to be a day of celebration. I often find myself praying to God that he blesses me with each of my future children to be born on June 25, the most special day of the year.

We haven't experienced a January 9 yet, the date of death. I am uneasy about how to handle this day and the emotions overwhelm me just thinking about it.

*

BELINDA LUNA
Belinda's full-term baby Elijah
died in utero in 2012 from trisomy 18

Unfortunately I haven't been able to formally honor my son's passing. Last year we wrote letters to him but I couldn't bring myself to put them in a balloon and set them free.

*

MELISSA MEAD
Melissa's 13-month-old son
William died in 2014 from sepsis

We haven't yet reached our first birthday without William, but it is fast approaching. William was born on my birthday, so the day is going to be extremely difficult. He was the most precious birthday present and was just meant to be.

For William's second birthday this year we have organized a balloon release using biodegradable balloons to mark his special day. There are friends, family and strangers coming that have been touched by William's story. William's favorite toy to play with was a balloon, he loved to hold the string and pull the balloon around to make lots of noise, so we are sending lots of balloons up to heaven for him to play with.

The anniversary of the day that William died was seventeen days after his first birthday and just eleven days before Christmas. It is going to be particularly hard. I think initially when he had just passed away, every hour that passes you look at the clock and imagine that twenty-four hours ago he was still alive....this time three days ago was the last time he ate breakfast. Sunday mornings are always difficult, and like clockwork I always seem to look at the clock at exactly 8:47 a.m. when William was pronounced dead.

The first anniversary this year will be as difficult as any other day, I still won't wake up with William; he will still be gone. I will simply be watching the clock knowing that this time last year was the moment I handed my baby over to the mortician.

*

SUSAN WILLIAMS
Susan's 2-month-old son
Tony died in 1987 from SIDS

The first few years were spent trying to get through the week, the whole week of the birthday, the whole week of the death date. Compassionate friends helped me so much with this anxiety. The actual date of both is just that: a date. I got through it. I will continue, for the rest of my life, to get through it. With that said, I started to be better to myself on these dates. I got a little selfish, because everyone kept telling me what I needed to do, which made me feel worse. So, I always took the day off work. I usually started the day either praying or going to Holy Mass. I made sure my other sons were with me, unless they were old enough to be in school. Sometimes, I put on the very few videos we had of Tony. I cried my eyes out, but I also smiled at the memories that the videos captured for Stu and I. Stu's parents gave us the video camera for Christmas two weeks before Tony was born. Ironic, huh? What a gift.

This is the ultimate gift Tony gave me on his two-year death date: I took the day off from school, and Zach and I spent the day together. Zach was three years-old, and I wish I could say he had a good day with his mother. I'm sure he doesn't remember it, and I'm fortunate that he doesn't. It must have sucked to be him that day. I literally cried the entire morning. He kept bringing me Kleenex from the bathroom and hugging me. Around noon I got a phone call. It was another school system that was looking for a music teacher. I told them that I currently was employed, but thank you for calling me. After I hung up the phone, I felt the urge to think about this opportunity. I never asked any questions. I immediately called back, and the woman told me that it never hurts to interview. Within three weeks my life had completely turned around. I spent the next twenty-five years in that system. Tony was behind that. I know the decision was made by me, but the urging came from him. That was one of the best decisions I made in my life.

Those twenty-five years were spent honoring Tony. I always knew he was beside me throughout those years. I taught in a school system that had a lot of poverty, neglect, and addiction problems with parents. It was tough to put up with that, when you have lost a child. Many nights I would come home and cry knowing all I could do was pray for some of my students. It really got to me. There were three times that I had to call the police because the parents never came to pick up their child from after-school choir. In addition, I had to remove the child from choir because of the neglect of their parent. Choir was the only activity these children had!

I paid a babysitter to watch my children "overtime" because they knew I would babysit their children for free. Most often, the children that I had to remove from choir due to parental neglect were my most talented students. My concern, love, and sorrow for these children cannot be measured.

81

Currently, since I have had these dates for twenty-eight years, I do a special surprise for someone on Tony's birthday. I might give someone a gift or surprise and sign it: with hugs and tons of love. Usually it is for someone going through a really tough time.

On Tony's death date, it's usually a day I'm praying, outside in nature, or sacrificing in some way for someone who needs help. This date is more difficult than Tony's birthday, so I might as well help someone because I'm going to focus on Tony's death and the circumstances that happened that particular day. If I'm busy and someone gets helped in some way, I can feel good about a smile that came from someone who needed it.

*

CHAPTER SEVEN

THE HOLIDAYS

The only predictable thing about grief is that it's unpredictable. - LYNDA CHELDELIN FELL

The holiday season comes around like clockwork, and for those in mourning, this time of year brings a kaleidoscope of emotions. If the grief is still fresh, the holidays can be downright raw. How do we navigate such a festive season that once held the promise of magical holiday memories?

*

DIANNA VAGIANOS ARMENTROUT
Dianna lost her newborn baby
Mary Rose in 2014 to trisomy 18

Holidays upset me. Mother's Day. Halloween. Christmas. I miss my daughter so much, and think of the possibilities of the other two pregnancies. How can I not be sad during the holidays? Where are all the sad people in the midst of the festivities and consumerism? The holidays remind me how much I miss my daughter, though I don't miss her more on these days. There seems to be less room for Mary Rose on the holidays than my ordinary days because people expect me to be happy and cheery. We are together with others and there are expectations to make memories with our loved ones, but what about the loved ones who died before any memories could be made?

Last Christmas, which was the second Christmas after Mary Rose, I bought chocolates as gifts and put them in her stocking. I gave them to my son and niece and nephew on Christmas morning. I don't know how I was alone in that moment, but the rest of the family was dispersed around the house. I cried as I mentioned my daughter's name, embracing my healthy and thriving son, niece and nephew. I don't want Mary Rose to be forgotten. I want her to be a part of the family and our traditions. It is particularly hard with our losses because we don't have a sense of the child's personality to remember. I want my children with me always, but especially on holidays and on milestones. I wept the day my son started church school. I cry at his birthday.

Where is my daughter? Where are my children whom I love? I light a tea candle near Mary Rose's picture, and remember her as I celebrate holidays with my living son and husband.

*

LINDA BATEMAN GOMEZ
Linda's 8-week-old son Chad
died in 1986 from SIDS

The holidays have gotten way better over the years. There is no question that the music, festivities, and the idea of spending time with family and friends can bring with it a terrible emptiness when someone special is missing. Especially when it is a child and even more so, if your loss is recent. When you lose an infant, you cannot help but think how they will never get to enjoy this wonderful time of year and you feel a sadness for those missed occasions.

Our family deals with holidays similar to how we deal with Chad's birthday. It is usually a trip to the cemetery and flowers. For Christmas I do hang an empty stocking with the others on the fireplace. When Chad first died the usual holiday joy was gone but we had two little girls, so while we may not have felt it in our hearts we were careful to not let Chad's death take the happiness from his sisters. We made the season as normal as possible for them.

Mother's Day is probably the hardest for me. Having lost my child and then three years later my mother, there is truly an extra heaviness for me. Christmas and Thanksgiving are also still sad, but nothing like the early years. Over the years the holidays, like all of the other things that seemed so overwhelming when I first lost Chad, were healed with time. There will always be an empty stocking and a heaviness in my heart of course, but the season is once again filled with laughter and joy.

*

MARY LEE CLAFLIN
Mary Lee's 2-month-old grandson Lane
died in 1998 from carbon monoxide poisoning

When Lane first died, I would go to the cemetery all the time, not just on special occasions. If I was feeling down or something was bothering me I would go sit and talk to him. Christmas was the hardest of all the holidays. We had just celebrated Lane's first Christmas with us at my house. We took pictures and had him sitting under the tree in his infant seat. For the first several years after, I would take a Christmas tree or flowers and have a conversation with him. Then I would say a prayer for him. I don't think I have ever gone there without crying after all these years. I kept remembering how tiny the casket was and how little he looked laying there. I miss him and always wondered what he would look like today. I was always looking into the future and saying, "What if…." and, "If only…" Since moving several hours away, I no longer go to the cemetery as much, but he is always in my heart.

*

ANNAH ELIZABETH
Annah Elizabeth's son Gavin Michael aspirated on his meconium
during delivery in 1990 and died 26 minutes following his birth

The earliest holidays were the hardest. We endured several Mother's Days and Father's Days without a child. Halloween.

Christmas. Valentine's Day. Easter. No silly costumes. No child for Santa's lap, no cheesy photo ops, and no little one's stocking to hang. Warren bought me one of those mechanical bunnies around the first Easter. I remember bawling because it reminded me of what I was missing. When Fave came along, I felt a little bit of initial guilt at being happy, but the presence of this child seemed to dull the pain of missing the first.

A year or two after we buried Gavin, Warren and I made seasonal, wooden decorations to put on his grave. I created the stencils, transferred them to wood, and then painted them after Warren carved them out. We had an Easter bunny reading a book, several Easter eggs, some spring flowers, a couple of Christmas stockings, and a Santa Claus. We keep all of these items in an oversized boot box that has its own place on a shelf in our closet.

For Gavin's birthday, we always buy a few balloons and some special spring decoration, since his special day falls on the heels of winter's end. We pull unwanted weeds from around his grave marker, we pad the empty space with pine needles, and set out the gifts we brought. On his twenty-first birthday we went to a special restaurant we'd never visited before and I had a chocolate raspberry martini in his honor.

We've participated in an Easter sunrise pageant for the past fourteen years. We come home to find the treasure the Easter bunny left behind, have breakfast, and then head to the cemetery before returning home for a nap or a rousing video game found in one of the baskets. Visiting Gavin is as much a part of our holiday traditions as the homemade pumpkin, apple, and pecan pies that grace our buffet, a staple in our family's celebrations. If Warren and I fail to mention that part of our day, one of the children will inevitably ask about when we're going.

One of my most special traditions, though, is how we form a circle around his stone. Hands held, we wonder aloud about things he might be doing in heaven, what toys he would have been playing with or, when he became of driving age, what kind of car he'd be driving. We take turns sending Gavin a special message. I've always believed that Gavin's spirit is with us wherever we are, so visiting the cemetery is more of a formality for us, but it is the tradition that my three living children have always known and it is one they've always remembered.

A few blocks from the cemetery, there's a little store that sells the best locally made ice cream and eggnog. They are always open Christmas Day. As my children grew older, we would stop to buy several half gallons of the frozen treats to top our after-dinner pie. While there, we'd also pick up a few lottery tickets for everyone to scratch off. When they were younger the kids knew they couldn't cash them in, but, oh, the delight once they became of age!

The other special part of these events is that we are creating memories with our loved one, even when he is not in this physical plane. Gavin has always been and will always be a part of these stories. It is a relationship that we have continued to develop, even in his absence. One of the most beautiful things I learned in my healing is that we can create new memories and carry on relationships with our loved ones after they are gone, it's just that they exist in ways we never expected.

*

NEISHA HART
Neisha's 6-month-old daughter
Brimley died in 2015 to SUID

The holidays are the worst time of the year. We were finally just getting to the point where we were making our own family traditions and I didn't want to do anything but spend time with my family. That is what made me the happiest. Halloween, Thanksgiving, and Christmas are still to come for this first year, and I find myself asking to pick up shifts at work so I won't have to make excuses to avoid family during these times. I don't want to see all my siblings opening presents with their children while I just sit there and watch. I feel like these feelings are going to remain until we have a another child of our own to unwrap gifts with again.

*

BELINDA LUNA
Belinda's full-term baby Elijah
died in utero in 2012 from trisomy 18

We were never able to spend any holidays with Elijah however there is always something missing: HIM! I have an ornament with his ultrasound picture that hangs on our tree every year.

*

MELISSA MEAD
Melissa's 13-month-old son
William died in 2014 from sepsis

I think all holidays are equally hard. I share my birthday with William, so now instead of being extra special our birthdays will now be fraught with grief. It doesn't feel like a day to celebrate, it is a day to share memories. But I do that every day.

Trying to find the energy to organize something special, which is what William deserves, is extremely difficult when you are consumed by despair.

Christmas will always be particularly difficult. William passed away eleven days before Christmas, so that first Christmas I spent at the Chapel of Rest, holding my baby and talking to him. I doesn't seem right to celebrate Christmas without him, when Christmas is all about him.

*

SUSAN WILLIAMS
Susan's 2-month-old son
Tony died in 1987 from SIDS

Tony died a week before Easter. The flowers were beautiful, I had my two sons, I had a job, and my life was going in the way I always pictured it! After Tony died I struggled with God. I remember screaming at HIM, "Why? Why? What did I do wrong?"

Growing up a cradle-Catholic I was destined for hell. The way I felt about God was hate. Everything I had been taught blew up in my face. I never thought I was a bad person. If you were a good person, you would be blessed by God. That day I feared God. I didn't understand why I was living. Everything I believed in just died with Tony. I must have done something so wrong to have God punish me so harshly. I was totally dumbfounded on what it could have been.

Right before Good Friday I was crying uncontrollably in the middle of the night. I heard the Virgin Mother say to me, "Susan, I did nothing wrong either, however my son, Jesus Christ was crucified in front of me." She stayed with me for a while and I felt her hug me until I was ready to understand what just happened to me. It took me quite a while to believe that she really came to comfort me. This changed my life.

Now I go to the Virgin Mary for all my sorrows. I can't say that my suffering and grief got better, but I can say that I know God did not take my son from me. I know that it was not for something I did wrong. That gave me comfort. After that locution from Our Lady I was able to heal. Holy Thursday, Good Friday and Easter have a special meaning for me. They are very holy and spiritual in my life. I was given a gift that I was unworthy of. Even when I was screaming at God, he loved me, like a mother or father would do with their own children.

Christmas was extremely hard on me the first years of grief. After I had Ben, it became easier to bear. I think Christmas is such a child's holiday. It's pretty tough on bereaved parents and grandparents. Even though we had Zach, we couldn't forget about Tony. It was another reminder that we would never be a complete family ever. Even after Ben came into our family, we were still not complete. We will never be complete until we are together in heaven. That will be the best gift I could ever receive. I'm sure that's how Our Lady feels right now. She is with her family in heaven and now she is joyful. That's what she wants for us as well.

I miss everything about you.
I miss the way you would always point your big toe up.
I miss the way you always pointed your finger,
even when there was nothing to point at.
I miss waking up before you and being impatient,
waiting for you to wake up.
I miss when you would get excited, tensing and pointing your feet.
I miss you giving them a little wiggle for extra excitement.
I miss the way you stood at the stair gate
posting balls from your ball pool into the kitchen.
I miss how you sat at the bottom of the stairs
waiting for daddy to take you for a shower.
I miss your gorgeous little bum.
I miss being able to squidge your gorgeous little bum.
I miss your smell, your intoxicating smell,
it was always the best in the morning.
I miss my morning fix.
I miss reading your nursery cards, what you'd eaten,
played with, what you'd achieved.
I miss picking you up from nursery,
to see your little face when you would catch a glimpse of me,
to see the emotion erupt on your face,
you would cry you were so overwhelmed.
I miss the way that mummy would pout her lips and huff for you to copy.
I miss being able to say "up," your little hands shot in the air
and we would have a cuddle.
I miss snuggling you into my chest and giving you milk before sleepies.
I will never forget that eye contact.
I miss not being able to lose myself in your big brown eyes.
I miss knowing that you're sleeping in the next room.
I miss hearing your faint snore.
I miss getting to work and finding the toys you'd put in my bag.
I miss putting your shoes on for the tenth time before nursery.
I miss pointing out your window before sleepies, watching the stars.
I miss your laugh.
I miss missing yesterday.
I miss knowing that there is a tomorrow.
I miss the way you made me feel.
You are the sun in my day,
the wind in my sky,
the waves in my ocean,
and the beat in my heart.
I miss you.
MELISSA MEAD

CHAPTER EIGHT

THE BELONGINGS

An angel, in the Book of Life, wrote down my baby's birth. Then whispered as he closed the book, "Too beautiful for Earth." - UNKNOWN

Our baby's belongings are a direct connection to what once was and what we desperately want back. They ARE what is left of our child until one day the smell has dissipated, the threads are bare, or we discover a need greater than our own. When does the time come to address the painful task of sorting our baby's memory-laden belongings, and how does one begin?

*

DIANNA VAGIANOS ARMENTROUT
Dianna lost her newborn baby
Mary Rose in 2014 to trisomy 18

I put my pregnancy clothes away right after I gave birth to Mary Rose. I recently went through my son's newborn things and my pregnancy clothes. I had such a feeling of despair when I looked at the maternity clothes so I gave most of them away to the veterans. I was able to feel some joy at my son's things remembering his birth instead of focusing on how I didn't know if Mary Rose would need them during my second pregnancy. I did keep one shirt and one pajama bottom that I wore a lot during pregnancy. I labored in the pajama pants and they have roses on them. They are in a memory box that I made to keep Mary Rose's few things. If there is another pregnancy I don't want to wear the clothes that I was so sad wearing before.

*

LINDA BATEMAN GOMEZ
Linda's 8-week-old son Chad
died in 1986 from SIDS

I still have all of Chad's belongings, including the bassinet he passed away in. After Chad died, well-meaning family and friends continued to push me to put his things away, but I wasn't ready. I didn't want help and I didn't want anyone to touch his things.

There was one family member who was especially pushy and, while well meaning, I felt far overstepped her bounds. Her actions were not helpful and it was my husband who intervened. It is really helpful if there is someone that you can go to should you not be strong enough at times to stand up to things you are not yet ready to deal with. I was blessed with both my husband and my mother understanding that I needed time and help, but not someone telling me what they wanted me to do.

Early on I felt comfort going into Chad's nursery where I could still hold his things and smell the baby smell on them. Then one day about six months after Chad had passed away, I went in by myself and started to pack his things. My husband was really surprised to see me doing this and asked if I needed help. I didn't though, I just cried and hugged his things as I would pack them. Each piece had a special meaning and memory. It was surprising how much stuff a tiny baby already had, as it filled several boxes. I left all of Chad's pictures and personal things up, but his clothing, blankets, and bedding I put away and placed in his closet. As time passed, I could never part with his things. Some of the boxes did get moved into the garage after a number of years, but I still have everything. They hold for me the few physical memories of Chad that I ever had.

Holding on to things is a personal choice and again, there is no right or wrong. Some people don't need to keep the belongings, or may donate them knowing that someone might benefit from them. For those like myself, they bring comfort. For another, they may bring up reminders that are still too painful. I think the important thing to remember is to do what is best for you and your family and on your own time. Don't feel rushed to make these decisions, especially if you are getting rid of things. Once they are gone they cannot be replaced. You will know when you are ready and what it is that you want to do. Something else to possibly consider is that a family member might want something. My mother for example wanted a T-shirt just so that she also had a small physical reminder. It made me happy to share that with her. Again, just another thing to possibly consider.

Chad is very much a presence in our home and always will be. His pictures are still up in the house, as are a few special things that I keep on my dresser and will until the day I die. These things, once so painful to see because they reminded me only of his loss, are now a sweet memory of him and bring me both comfort and a smile.

*

KARI BROWN
Kari's 2-year-old daughter Dominique (Deedee)
died in 2014 from obstructive sleep apnea

Handling Dominique's belongings was hard, but we had to move three months after she passed. We packed everything else first, and let her room for last. It was extremely difficult, and I could not get through even one hour of packing without crying. It felt as if I was packing her memories away. We were moving in with Brandon's step-brother, so we could not bring much and had to keep most of our belongings in storage. I hated the idea of leaving Dominique's things in storage; it felt like they should be with us, in the open.

A lot of emotions came up: anger, bitterness, heartbreak and especially sadness. We packed things that she loved or never had a chance to wear. A few things were picked out that we could bring with us: a couple of her favorite clothing items she loved to wear, and a couple of favorite toys that we wanted to keep close to us. After we moved into our own apartment, we unpacked some of her belongings such as a few toys and more clothing items that we could hang next to ours. We moved into a one-bedroom apartment so we didn't have space for her crib or other large furniture. But having her items around the apartment like her beanbag, feeding utensils (bowls, bottles, silverware) and her trunk of toys helped to ease our ache of her absence. We have always talked about moving into a house and setting up her room the way it was before. It may sound crazy, but it reminds us that we are still parents.

*

MARY LEE CLAFLIN
Mary Lee's 2-month-old grandson Lane
died in 1998 from carbon monoxide poisoning

When we came home that night from the hospital, people were coming over to bring food and visit with us. My son told us to start cleaning up the living room. He wanted the bassinet put in the nursery and the bottles in the kitchen out of sight. He did not want people to come in and see anything that had to do with Lane. We moved everything into the nursery and closed the door. I don't know how long it took my daughter-in-law to put Lane's clothes and other articles away. Since there was a lawsuit, the lawyer took the clothes and diaper bag that was with Lane when he died. Later they gave the articles to my son. He stopped by my house on the way home and said I could look in the bag and see if I wanted anything. I took the tiny baby socks that Lane had on when he was taken to the hospital. I still have these socks and will give them to his mother one day. About once a year I go through a special box of Lane's that holds all the cards, notes, donation letters and see these socks. It still makes my heart hurt and tears come to my eyes.

*
ANNAH ELIZABETH
Annah Elizabeth's son Gavin Michael aspirated on his meconium during delivery in 1990 and died 26 minutes following his birth

I'm not sure where it came from, but while I was in the hospital following Gavin's death someone brought me a large box. One of my strongest memories is of me holding that square clothing container on my lap as the staff person wheeled me to the front door of the hospital, where my husband waited with the car, the one with the baby carrier we'd painstakingly secured in the back seat, well in advance of our baby's arrival.

My son's entire life seemed to be packed into a piece of mass-produced cardboard: his hospital blanket and hand-knitted hat, the paper measuring tape that recorded his birth statistics, the bassinet card, the many condolences and the two Mother's Day cards friends and family sent. I later added copies of the love letters and the farewell letters Warren and I wrote before Gavin's funeral. I also added the floral tags, the VCR tape of his only ultrasound, the few photos his nurses took of him, the funeral guest registry, the funeral bulletin, the scraps of paper I'd recorded my contractions on, and the photos Warren and I took with him at the funeral home.

Twenty-five years after Gavin's birth, those treasures are preserved in that same box, which I now keep in a fireproof safe.

I had so many items that I ended up filling a large, plastic, handled-shopping bag with Gavin's other belongings: photos from my pregnancy, special items from my baby shower, another baby book, the many other condolence cards and special notes we received from family, friends, and even a few strangers, the baptismal jacket I hadn't put on Gavin because I chose to send him off in the crocheted sweater my mother-in-law had made especially for him.

My boss and I were pregnant at the same time, our boys born two weeks apart. We shared McDonald's buttered biscuits in the mornings, chocolate confections whenever the urge struck, as well as our hopes and fears. And we, along with our spouses, finished out our pregnancies in the same Lamaze group. It was in one of our final birthing classes that our instructor ended the session with a task none of us expected. "I know you're all in happy places with happy times ahead," she began, "but I would like you to ponder something—what you would do if something happened to the baby? I know it's not anything you want to think about but you should really spend a minute or two discussing it," she finished.

"What would you do if something happened to the baby?" I asked Warren on the way home. "I don't know," he replied. "You?" "I don't know either," I said. We didn't talk about it again. Until we had to.

Like all of the other pregnancy related matters my pregnant pal and I shared, we shared our experiences around that turn of topic. She told me that she and her husband had also considered that question on their drive home. "I told him if something happened I didn't want him to do anything with the nursery; I would want to come home to it just the way I've prepared it," she said.

I was grateful to have that foresight and equally thankful to have the freshly washed bedding to cuddle with and the mobile's music to listen to as I grieved, dreamed, and sometimes fell asleep in the antique rocker at the foot of Gavin's crib.

I ended up using the nursery items for each of my three children to come. Like life, the threads and fibers of those belongings bear the marks of good and bad, happy and sad, laughter and tears. For me, all these years later, they are more like symbols, little tangible objects that Gavin lived. Those things, however, are nothing more than fabricated products. One of the truths I've always told my children and my students is that material possessions come and go...they are expendable, but our relationships are forever. The bond I have with my son is eternal. Nothing can take that away.

Even though I occasionally have fleeting moments of longing—like when Gavin's would-be playmate proposed to his girlfriend, when I watched those two stand at the altar and exchange their vows, and when I helped them welcome their own first child—I am now able to celebrate the life I had with my son and the one I continue to have with him. It is a connection independent of stuff; one that is filled to brimming in a form that is far different from that which I'd ever expected, envisioned and imagined.

*

NEISHA HART
Neisha's 6-month-old daughter
Brimley died in 2015 to SUID

At first we just shut the door to the nursery and pretended it wasn't there. I was afraid to go in there by myself or even be home alone at night in all honesty. Almost a year later, and I still get those feelings. When we felt comfortable enough to go in there, we gathered up things that we knew people would want and made sure everyone had a keepsake to remember our daughter by. At one point, every piece of clothing came out of the dresser and the closet and laid just in piles on the floor. It was a disaster in there! I went to the store and bought ten clear tubs to sort and organize different sizes by. Once we found out we were pregnant again, things were kicked into high gear and everything was neatly put away.

We kept Brimley's main everyday items, like her activity bouncer, bumbo and highchair, out for a while until we finally felt comfortable living our daily lives without touching or staring at these items as everyday reminders of what we are missing. At one point, I asked my dad if he would take the activity bouncer to the storage unit just so it was out of the way. But by the time he was getting around to doing it, I had changed my mind. I needed it here with us. I needed it in the living room in front of the TV so I didn't feel like something was missing from us, even though it was.

*

MELISSA MEAD
Melissa's 13-month-old son
William died in 2014 from sepsis

As I write this, it has been ten months since we lost our beautiful boy. Every item of William's things are exactly where they were before he died. As William passed away at home, in his bed, his bedding was moved by the paramedics. When they pronounced him dead, they told us we needed to go to the hospital and they began to wrap William in a towel that was nearby. I refused and told them not to touch William, he was my baby. I curled up on the floor next to him, my cheek pressed against his, my hand on his other cheek and I begged him to wake up. I pleaded with him to wake up, but he didn't. I was reminded that we needed to go to the hospital, so I got his fluffy blanket out of his wardrobe. I wrapped him up and carried him every step of the way. Ten months on, the towel that the paramedics originally used to wrap William in, albeit for only a few seconds, still lays in his bedroom. I can't move it, let alone use it.

I am very possessive over William's things, his coat still hangs on his peg, his sippy cup lays where he left it in his cot, his toys are still in the front room, and his rubber ducks still sit on the side of the bath. Both William's dad and I don't want to move any of William's things. He's still part of our family, his car seat is still in the car. We have no reason to move it, so simply, we don't.

The only things that have been moved are the clothes William wore those last few days. I had done all the washing, as we were due to go on holiday two days after William died, and these were the few items that really held his strawberry sweet smell. His favorite reindeer teddy and his little rabbit are all sealed in a vacuum bag so that when I need to I can take them out and hold them and breathe in their smell.

William had just taken his first independent steps a few days before he passed away. I had bought him a beautiful pair of leather shoes that would give him support. I had a lovely box frame made for those shoes, and they hang on the wall. Seeing William's belongings really hurts but it's bittersweet, they hold so many beautiful memories as well.

*

SUSAN WILLIAMS
Susan's 2-month-old son
Tony died in 1987 from SIDS

The grandparents tried to protect Stu and I so much that they started the process of washing clothes and insisting we move things immediately. Looking back, they were just doing what parents do for their children. They were hurting so bad, and they wanted to help us in any way they could. What they did not know is how much I needed to smell those clothes after Tony died. I needed to remember his scent. I needed to keep some of those clothes without them being washed of my son's last hours on earth. How could they know that? How could I tell them that they took this away from me without hurting them more?

The crib and other items were quickly put away as well. This all took place as we were preparing for the funeral. I needed time to process what just happened to me, and removing all Tony's belongings was upsetting me. I remember getting upset about it in front of a group of family members that had come over to comfort me. I was an emotional time bomb. I hurt more knowing that I had hurt someone else's feelings, so I continued to allow friends and family to "think" they were helping me. Usually, I allowed them to do whatever they felt they needed to do. I just didn't have the energy to fight any battles. I was fighting to breathe. Every moment was difficult to handle. What I really wanted was everyone to leave me alone in my sorrow, but that was not reality. They hurt too. I couldn't help them, and unfortunately they couldn't help me either.

Eighteen years later, when Tony would have graduated from high school, I felt the urge to take out all the baby cards, baptism cards, and the few keepsakes I had stored away. I really struggled that year, knowing I missed his whole childhood. It occurred to me that these items could be put in a scrapbook for me. I took some scrapbook classes, and I grieved through the childhood I missed with my son. As difficult as this was, it was a very huge milestone for me. I took my time, and created a gift for myself on his graduation.

I took my scrapbook to a Compassionate Friends meeting and shared my gift with the members. It encouraged some others to do the same thing. Most of the members brought in their huge scrapbooks full of memories that gave them peace and reminders of their many years with their deceased children. Unfortunately, my scrapbook is very small. It is a constant reminder of how little time I had with my son.

Sometimes, I get jealous of the time the other members had with their children. I continue to feel robbed of his entire childhood. The only time I feel guilty of this emotion is when a mother and father come into a Compassionate Friends meeting and tell me about their stillborn child. In my opinion, their loss is even greater. This is my personal opinion. I try not to compare losses. This is not a competition, but the parents of stillborn children have less in their scrapbook than me. The parents of stillborn children remind me that every moment I had with Tony was a gift. Even if it was only ten weeks. It was longer than some parents had with their children.

*

CHAPTER NINE

THE DARKNESS

How very quietly you tiptoed into our world, silently, only a moment you stayed. But what an imprint your footprints have left upon our hearts.
-UNKNOWN

Suicidal thoughts are not uncommon in the immediate aftermath of profound loss, yet few readily admit it for fear of being judged or condemned. While there would be no rainbow without the rain, where do we find the energy to fight the storm?

*

DIANNA VAGIANOS ARMENTROUT
Dianna lost her newborn baby
Mary Rose in 2014 to trisomy 18

After Mary Rose's diagnosis, I did think about throwing myself down a cliff near my house when I was walking with my son. It was one moment and it passed. I shared this thought with my therapist and midwife and they were both concerned, but they saw that I was functioning and eating and taking care of my son. I realized even in my grief and shock that I had so many blessings in my life, even with the trisomy 18 diagnosis. I love my family. I want my family. I breathed through small miracles in each moment as my mentor, Sister Evelyn, of Mount St. Mary's Abbey taught me when my aunt was terminally sick. Sister Evelyn told me to look for the small miracles all around me in the face of my aunt's decline. They were there all along. I had to look for them.

After Mary Rose's death, I wanted the earth to take me into her. This was a visceral and physical feeling, but I had no desire to take my life. I vowed that I would help others with my experience and live a life of service. God knows why my daughter was chosen to have a body with trisomy 18. She might not be in an earthly body, but her life continues in other dimensions.

*

LINDA BATEMAN GOMEZ
Linda's 8-week-old son Chad
died in 1986 from SIDS

After Chad died, I did just want to die. The pain was so overwhelming and unbearable that I didn't think it was even possible to go on with life in that much pain.

While I wanted to make the pain stop, I'm not sure suicide is what I could call it, as I never thought about a way or had a plan to actually do anything. I remember telling my husband how I wish I would die to stop the pain of my broken heart. He said he knew what I meant and his recognition of that was actually a surprise for me. He and I handled things very differently, I was very emotional and had no problem showing it. He was much more controlled, so when he said he understood, I realized that although he was not as open and emotional about verbalizing his feelings, he still felt the same intense pain that I was feeling.

While we were both so sad and hurting so much, and both thought the pain was unbearable, we also recognized suicide was never an option. I think having two other children and knowing the kind of pain it would cause for others, especially our children and our parents, made considering actually doing something to ourselves unthinkable. We just let time start to heal us, as we all know it does. Though it sometimes seems like it is never going to happen, it will. If it feels like you can't go on, you can! You just have to hold on, it will get better, I promise. No matter how dark it seems, the light will come.

*

KARI BROWN
Kari's 2-year-old daughter Dominique (Deedee) died in 2014 from obstructive sleep apnea

I have had thoughts of suicide when my daughter passed, but I couldn't do that to my mother. She had already lost her husband and an infant years before, and now a granddaughter. I mentioned my thoughts of suicide to a couple of very close friends, but had no intention of following through with it. I just wanted to die so that I could be with Dominique again. I wanted to die so that I wouldn't have to feel this daily heartbreak, and the occasional bitterness I feel when seeing other parents with their children.

But instead of thinking more about suicide, I thought about what I could do. I could help by sharing my story with others and offering advice when asked. I found that by sharing my experience, I pass on Dominique's light and love to new people who have never met her. So I feel proud to be able to turn pain into something positive, and help others by sharing what Dominique taught me.

*

MARY LEE CLAFLIN
Mary Lee's 2-month-old grandson Lane died in 1998 from carbon monoxide poisoning

As Lane's grandmother, I did not have thoughts of suicide. I had gone through a hurtful divorce several years prior and I did have suicidal thoughts at that time and was put in a psychiatric hospital for several days. I started going to a therapist for help. Very shortly after Lane was buried I went back into counseling. I recognized sad and depressed, it was a friend of mine. Even with counseling I never got over the thought that I caused Lane's death by recommending the sitter. Neither my son nor daughter-in-law ever made me feel like it was my fault. This helped me to work through this loss.

*

ANNAH ELIZABETH
Annah Elizabeth's son Gavin Michael aspirated on his meconium during delivery in 1990 and died 26 minutes following his birth

This is a simple, yet equally complicated question. The simple answer is "yes," I thought about suicide after my son's death. The more complicated answer is that I had also been dealing with a long, undiagnosed depression that had also contributed to suicidal thoughts I'd had in my teen years. In the five year span following Gavin's death I also experienced two miscarriages and two more complicated pregnancies that ended in successful births.

My husband and I were young parents who were each grieving and celebrating differently. We were trying to navigate a family business and realizing the differences in our thought processes about most everything, including parenting, business practices, and the roles other relationships should play in our own little family. My body was tired, stretched out and stressed beyond recognition. On a particularly grueling night it all came to a head. Alcohol and I had always had a tenuous time of it; sometimes I'd be the life of a party after a few drinks and other times my mood swings would turn the merriment into a nightmare. Not knowing about the depression, I figured the alcohol was fully responsible for the outbursts and had chosen to either abstain from legal beverages or to limit my consumption to the occasional one or two beers.

I began writing in a journal on May 30, 1995, a few short days following one of the last times I'd ever fall into that state of suicidal drunkenness again. I found a compatible therapist and began the grueling task of tapping into my long-standing depression and undoing the many forms of dysfunctional thinking it had caused. Frequent thoughts of suicide had become one of those side effects. I remember telling my therapist that I'd figured out a way to take my life but make it look like an accident, an important detail because I didn't want my living children to have to face the future stigma. Counselor Hank responded with this pearl of wisdom, "If you really wanted to be dead, Annah, you'd be dead by now." He couldn't have been any closer to the truth, for what I really wanted was for the pain to go away so that I could truly live.

There was a point in all of this when I realized that I couldn't take my own life so I switched from plotting to pleading with God. This was one of my prayers: "God please take me tonight. I can't endure the pain. Everyone says You aren't a cruel God. They say You don't give us more than we can handle. You must know my agony; I can't bear any more. You know I can't bring myself to end my own life. Please, God, have mercy. End my suffering."

I distinctly remember that day. Gavin came to me that night. He was dressed in white shorts with suspenders and a white top, a sort of baptismal outfit. "I'm okay, Mommy," he said, "You need to stay there; my brother and sister need you."

That event created a turning point for me, a foundation that I've continued to build upon. Immediately, it gave me something to hold on to, something to help me get through each day. It gave me hope and it helped me consider my son's spirit in a whole new light and it provided me a different sort of promise.

*

NEISHA HART
Neisha's 6-month-old daughter
Brimley died in 2015 to SUID

I think everyone who experiences a loss of some sort has a moment of weakness and thinks about what it would be like to not live with the daily pain and hurt anymore. I don't think I ever had thought of committing the act of suicide, but I often catch myself thinking about how I am not afraid to die anymore. One of my top fears I used to have was the fear of dying, and now that no longer bothers me at all. I catch myself daydreaming about getting into an

105

accident or being in an altercation like a robbery, and not being afraid to die, almost thankful that the robber or accident would reunite me with my children that I seldom see in my dreams. In a way, I'm sure that is along the same brainwave lengths as suicide, but I would never want to put my parents through what I am going though. I would rather be the one who takes the brunt of the hurt and anger over them any day.

*

MELISSA MEAD
Melissa's 13-month-old son
William died in 2014 from sepsis

For me, suicide is not about dying, it is about starting my life again with William. It's not about killing myself, but going to sleep and waking up with William. Before William died I had no idea what suicidal thoughts were or how they manifested. Seven weeks after William died, I tried to commit suicide. It was only because William's dad found me that I survived. I was, of course, admitted to the hospital and I had to undergo a mental health assessment. I have struggled with my mental health ever since.

It is very hard for people to understand what being suicidal feels like: to not feel like part of the world that is going on around you, to feel as though you exist in a fishbowl. To know that I can commit suicide is the only reason I make it through today. Suicide is part of my care plan, and I remain high risk. But knowing that I can end this existence tomorrow means that I don't have to do it today, and of course it's always "today." When I want to make my choice, I will. My mum said to me that to take my life is to be selfish. But let me ask you, those of you who haven't felt suicidal, is it not selfish to ask me to live a life I don't want to live just to save your feelings and not compound your pain?

I laid down, knowing that I had overdosed, and was waiting to drift off. It was about thirteen minutes, and was the most peaceful time I had felt since William died. I held his precious reindeer teddy, I looked at his photo, and I said, "Mummy will be with you soon." I have never been more disappointed when I was woken up by paramedics. Whilst they were taking me down the stairs, I asked my mum to look after William, to make sure that he was okay. For those moments, I didn't know. All over again to wake up in the morning and to relive this nightmare is torture. People assume that those who feel this way can just snap out of it. But you can't, it is something you live with. Living two parallel worlds is the hardest.

So if it wasn't for suicide, I would have killed myself by now. Suicide is my safety net. I didn't choose this, I didn't choose to feel like this. It is not something I can change. I fear tomorrow, knowing tomorrow is going to feel and be exactly the same as today. Time doesn't heal but only serves to widen the gap from the last time that I held my darling boy. As day slips away into night, I slip further away from William. So for me suicide isn't something I have felt, it's not something you overcome. It's something you live with.

*

SUSAN WILLIAMS
Susan's 2-month-old son
Tony died in 1987 from SIDS

Have I thought of suicide? Absolutely! I could never kill myself knowing that my parents would have to go through what I was going through at the time. The first few years I had many days that I knew death would be a relief from my gut-wrenching sorrow.

I enjoy wine and beer, so I tried to stay away from it. I knew I could easily drink myself to passing out. Thinking back, Zach was my reason for hope. I had to be the best mom I could for him. I was barely functioning, but he got me out of bed in the morning with, "Mommy, I'm up now."

*

What kind of mother has no child?
There are so, so many of us who have lived this truth,
this nagging question.
This is the kind of mother I was and am,
that you and our other grieving mothers are:
We are the women who longed for a child since we were young ourselves...
We are the women who swore we wanted no part of parenting
and somehow found ourselves with child; some of us embraced
this new life while others of us lament...something...
We are the women whose bodies bulged early or late,
whose breasts swelled and ached in preparation and then spilled over
when there was no mouth to release the stored up nourishment...
We are the women who laughed when we saw our friend's infant smile
as he passed gas and we dreamed when we spotted a toddler taking her
first steps...
Some of us plotted and planned a nursery while others plugged away,
bellies bulging, in the day-to-day grind...
We are the women whose children left their physical,
earthly form far earlier than we expected...
...the humans who plead with Gods to reveal the whys even after
we realize that sometimes the only explanation is simply Because it is...
...the beings who beg for forgiveness even when there is nothing to
forgive...
...and the souls who love, as I used to say to my three living children:
"Always, forever, and no matter what."
We love, Journeyer; we love so fully our bodies split with pride
and shame and joy and fear and hope...
Split wide open, sometimes...
Where this is great pain there is an even greater love.
ANNAH ELIZABETH

*

CHAPTER TEN

THE FRIENDS

Remember, you don't need a certain number of friends, just a number of friends you can be certain of. -UNKNOWN

When we are mourning, some of our friendships undergo transitions. Some bonds remain steady, dependable and faithful. Some we sever by choice. And, perhaps unexpectedly, new friends enter our life, bringing renewed hope rich with possibilities. How did your loss affect your friendships?

*

DIANNA VAGIANOS ARMENTROUT
Dianna lost her newborn baby
Mary Rose in 2014 to trisomy 18

Pregnant women and newborns continue to be a trauma trigger for me. My dear friend Paula is pregnant. She has the same due date I had with my October pregnancy. I saw her recently and it was hard. Paula was infertile and this is her first pregnancy. I am not jealous of her joy, but I feel my own empty body, although I have been ambivalent about trying to get pregnant again. My pregnancy was a time of great stress and grief. When I see pregnant women I remember that not-joy. Newborns also trigger my trauma of holding my dead baby in my arms. I get so upset every time I see a newborn and no one seems to notice or care. Our fragmented culture and lack of community is disheartening. There are times when I avoid public gatherings because I can't face pregnant women or newborns. My mentor Cubby LaHood, who cofounded Isaiah's Promise, the nonprofit that supports families carrying to term after a life-limiting diagnosis, didn't go near newborns for two years after her son Francis died the day he was born.

I often stay by myself rather than socialize with pregnant women. This has not lessened over time, perhaps because I had two miscarriages after my newborn died. I need to keep myself safe, and trauma triggers take a few days to wear off. I feel so raw as I walk around and move forward.

*

LINDA BATEMAN GOMEZ
Linda's 8-week-old son Chad
died in 1986 from SIDS

When Chad died, I was thirty-one years old. At that time, many of our friends were also having children. The children were friends and in many cases we did things together as families, like play dates or pizza nights. The truth is, it was very hard for me and for them, especially right after Chad died. The friends didn't know what to do or say and being around other infants was terrible for me. I didn't even like to go to the grocery store because seeing mothers with babies was so painful. I avoided places where I knew I would see this because that was what I needed to do for me at the time. The odd thing was that I had such a desire to hold an infant. Although I did try it early on with a friend's baby, it did not bring me the comfort I was hoping for. For the most part, like with many other issues, I found that time was once again the biggest healer.

Initially, I didn't spend a lot of time in person with the friends who had babies the same age as Chad, but we maintained the friendship by chatting on the phone. I suspect now, with social media there would be other ways to do that, but back then it was pretty much the telephone. It was being together in person and seeing the babies that was hard, but the friendships offered support and a kind voice or ear and that was really helpful.

As time passed, and I got stronger, we did get together again and it was fine. The only setbacks were things like the baby birthdays and other reminders of an important date in a child's life - starting school, graduations, etc. Even today, as these milestones happen for friends who had children at the same time, I am always reminded of a special life event that I am missing with Chad. These times are really bittersweet. While they still ring as a lost reminder for me, I am happy for my friends and I do enjoy celebrating these special occasions with them. They stood by me when I needed them and I celebrate with them now. True friends that stick with you in the worst of times are hard to find. I am blessed to have such wonderful people in my life.

*

MARY LEE CLAFLIN
Mary Lee's 2-month-old grandson Lane
died in 1998 from carbon monoxide poisoning

I had a very difficult time seeing people with babies. When they would baptize them at church, it hurt so much that I would get up and leave. I knew I would start crying. If a friend of mine had pictures to show me of their new grandbaby, it took all I could to say, "Yes, he/she is beautiful." I did not want to hear about when the baby rolled over, first smile, or making cute noises. That hurt and reinforced what I was missing as a grandmother. The lady at the church who recommended the sitter would see me and walk the other way. I always felt like she thought I blamed her. We never did talk like we did prior to Lane's death.

*
ANNAH ELIZABETH
Annah Elizabeth's son Gavin Michael aspirated on his meconium
during delivery in 1990 and died 26 minutes following his birth

Given the fact that my son died twenty-six minutes following his birth, I never really had a chance to develop friendships with other new parents. That said, I did experience conflict following Gavin's death.

My boss and I were pregnant at the same time. Our boys were born two weeks apart. Whereas my pregnancy went on without a single glitch until delivery, my employer—who was also a good friend I referred to as my pregnant pal—experienced many complications. We shared food cravings and sweet indulgences, name and nursery ideas, baby movements, our fears and joys, and sat through the same Lamaze lessons.

To this day I remember where I was, sitting at the desk in the corner of the office, when the call came. My eyes misted with happy tears as I listened to the baby's stats. It's definitely a boy. Weight. Length. Baby and Mom are fine. I was overwhelmed with gladness for her and her husband, a couple who had tried for nine long years to have a baby. Two weeks later I was equally torn apart by the tragedy of my son's death.

My sister, who lived some five hundred miles away, gave birth to my niece two weeks and a day after Gavin died. Our lives had taken us in different directions and though there has always been a sisterly bond, we weren't sharing those daily details, dread, and delights that my pregnant pal and I had. I have this memory of my mother phoning to tell me my sister's good news and suggesting I give her a call. I remember thinking that I didn't want to…that I couldn't…I just had a hard time feeling happy for her. I went on to beat myself up over that lack of joy for many years to come. Of course those ambivalent feelings eventually passed and I was able to think of my sister's family and my niece with joy, but it did take a little time.

Roughly four weeks following my sister's delivery, I started phasing back into work. The cesarean section allowed me an eight-week disability leave for recovery, but I was going stir crazy at home, so I begged my boss to let me do some of the non-time-sensitive paperwork each week. It was the type of pencil pushing that could be done anywhere, so I started out doing most of it at home, where I could put it off until later if I had a sudden outpouring of grief. By the time those two months had passed, I transitioned back to full-time hours.

My pregnant pal was more protective of my emotions than I was. Even though her in-laws babysat in a house behind the business, she tried to be thoughtful about bringing her son around me. I can honestly say, though, that seeing him and holding him brought me more comfort than pain. Yes, that sense of void was there, as was the longing for something different from what I had, but being included made me feel less isolated, less tarnished, less of a failure.

*

RENEE FORD-ROMERO
Renee's son Diego was stillborn due
to an undiagnosed cardiac fibroma in 2014

For the longest time I ran the other way at the sight of a pregnant woman, a baby, anything baby-related really. I felt that as a Christian, I wasn't supposed to be sad too long, or give the impression that I'm not grateful for the daughter I have. I find myself saying it too, like it's going to take away the longing for my babies. These are the kinds of things no human being can help you with. There is no appropriate length of time to grieve; there is no magic number of pregnancy announcements or baby commercials, and then suddenly you're healed. God allows me to grieve, just not stay in it.

Who knew that accidentally finding yourself in the baby section in Target or sitting in the obstetrician's waiting room could set off an emotional volcano? I have a monthly reminder of exactly how un-pregnant I am and, although sometimes it stirs up memories and I need a good cry, as a Christian I always have peace; the kind of peace that other people don't understand. The kind of peace no human being can give you. This kind of peace: *"And the peace of God, which transcends all understanding, will guard your hearts and your minds in Christ Jesus* (Philippians 4:7).

I attended a gender reveal party just a few weeks after I lost my son. This sweet, young couple was so excited, and something in me just wanted a piece of that. At the last minute though, I had second thoughts. I wasn't sure I could keep it together. Yet I attended, and it was amazing! It was so healing to see friends and family gathered to celebrate the creation of this little princess (pink balloons, it was a girl!). That sacrifice, the decision to choose joy over sadness, had lasting effects.

God has allowed a special spiritual connection with women in my circle who are pregnant or trying to conceive. He prompts me to pray about a young couple. and then the announcement comes. He prompts me to pray about a complicated pregnancy, and then the loss occurs. He prepares me to spread joy and comfort to those who need it.

He sent me a dream about one of my very best friends; that was terrifying! I dreamt that I was asking my boss for time off because my friend has passed away during childbirth, and her husband needed help with the baby. Although I've never revealed the details of the dream, I did tell my friend that I knew she was pregnant or would be soon, I just knew. She conceived the following month and I believe God showed me that the enemy would try to take her so that I could war on her behalf in the spiritual realm during her pregnancy. The day of her beautiful son's birth, we almost lost her. It felt like my nightmare was unfolding for real, but God healed her. She has experienced multiple losses and has overcome many obstacles in her health. She's the victory story, the miracle and I'm so grateful to be His witness!

*

NEISHA HART
Neisha's 6-month-old daughter
Brimley died in 2015 to SUID

I'm not sure if my loss affected my friendship with other parents. I have friends who have babies close in age to mine but was never super close to them where we hung out on a regular basis. The only time I ever feel it affecting me is when I am around my siblings. My dad's current wife has three children, plus me totals four. Each of us had a baby within a year of each other. This affects me because I should have my child there doing the same things at a family get-together or holiday party. The only other time I notice it affecting me is when I see someone announce that they are pregnant. I get real strong feelings of jealousy that it makes me upset with myself.

*

MELISSA MEAD
Melissa's 13-month-old son
William died in 2014 from sepsis

I didn't have many friends with young children, and initially it didn't bother me seeing other young children in the supermarket or at the doctors. It affects me more now, ten months down the line, than it did in those first few months. Why? Because in those initial months, I was consumed by shock. As time passes, although my mind remains foggy, I function better. When I see young children now, I imagine them to be William. I am jealous that those parents get to show their children the beach, chase after them in the supermarket, and get to see them every day. I am filled with sadness and despair when I see children the same age as William, knowing that his future and our future have been taken away.

My friend was pregnant when she came to William's funeral. I didn't know, and she was worried to tell me. But I was so happy for her. It doesn't make me feel bad, it doesn't fill me with envy but it does show me constantly what I'm missing out on. Knowing that they will get to a point where their little boy will be older than what William was when he died, does hurt. It makes me sick to know that at some point I will not know what William would have looked like. We're approaching William's second birthday, which is also my birthday, and I can imagine what a two-year-old William would look like. But when we get to ten years old, sixteen years old, or what William would look like as a man, I will never know, and it hurts so much.

*

SUSAN WILLIAMS
Susan's 2-month-old son
Tony died in 1987 from SIDS

Since Tony died at the babysitter's home, my relationships with all parents changed immediately. The babysitter had to go through an investigation of her childcare home. She was encouraged not to talk to me because of liability issues. My support system had been the parents of the children in this home, as well as my babysitter. I'm sure these parents had to find other childcare immediately. I do not know the specifics of what happened to this babysitter, but I can't imagine the horror she went through. She eventually gave up her profession. What a horrible loss for her. She had a good childcare service, and she had wonderful parents with wonderful kids whom she thought of as her own. My children were also thought of as her own. Her husband and two children went through a nightmare just like my family did. We could not talk to each other because of the complicated and sensitive issues that happened, unfortunately, at her house.

At the time of Tony's death, my best friends had children close to the ages of my children. It made it convenient if any of us needed to have a playdate or help with carpooling to nursery school. They all tried so hard to help me get back to normal after Tony died. They had no idea that I would never be the same ever again.

116

The more I put my "normal mask" on, the worse I became. I needed someone to hear my story over and over again. They really tried so hard to be tolerant of me, but I felt their anxiety when I was invited to be part of the group. Eventually, I wasn't invited very often. I totally understood, but it devastated me. I felt like a victim all over again. I realized that they needed to be joyful, like I used to be when my child was alive. I brought them to a place they were getting tired of going. Eventually, the friends stopped calling and I was totally alone.

Looking back, it wasn't anyone's fault. All my friends were in their middle twenties, starting their families, and they were scared that the same thing could happen to them. It happened to their good friend, and it was too close to home for them. I do see these people occasionally, and it still hurts me emotionally. It would have made a huge difference in my life if they had stayed by my side through the worst time of my life. Instead, I had to learn compassion the hard way: by learning what NOT to do when your friend loses a child.

Twenty-eight years later, I know these people were not the friends I thought they were. I have had the privilege of seeing what good friends look like. After I started going to Compassionate Friends meetings, I observed some bereaved parents had friends that accompanied them to the meetings for support. I saw what a good friend looks like. A good friend is someone who does not judge, or expect you to get back to "normal." It's someone who encourages you to do the best you can at any time. No judgment, just hugs, love, and lots of prayers. Good friends accompany you to a meeting. They drive you there and cry with you. They drive you home because your eyes are red and dry from crying for yourself and others who have lost children. Yes, you will cry too. But, because you are a good friend, you suffer too. Trust me, you will never feel the loss that a bereaved parent feels unless you are a bereaved parent.

Good friends watch you suffer, so they suffer too. The love of a good friend can soothe a broken heart. I have some friends that have comforted my broken heart. Every so often, the scab comes off, and they need to comfort me again. And they do. I am blessed!

*

CHAPTER ELEVEN

THE RELATIONSHIPS

Each new life, no matter how brief, forever changes
the world. -UNKNOWN

For many of us, familial relationships are the cornerstones that help us stay sane; they keep us laughing, learning, and loving. We speak one another's language and finish one another's sentences. Sometimes, however, loss touches us in different ways. What family relations, if any, were impacted by the loss of your baby?

*

DIANNA VAGIANOS ARMENTROUT
Dianna lost her newborn baby
Mary Rose in 2014 to trisomy 18

My husband and I had very different responses to our grief over Mary Rose's condition and death. There was no place where I could step away from the reality of trisomy 18. I could not separate my body from Mary Rose and, once she was born, my postpartum body physically wanted its newborn. I have never grieved so physically for so long. My husband has a good and open heart, but he is able to compartmentalize and stay busy. Tim tried to ignore Mary Rose's diagnosis before she was born. I handled most of the medical and birth planning. Where I was nearly paralyzed by shock after Mary Rose died, my husband stayed home from work for one week and then got busy. I needed to feel my pain, but he opened himself up to his grief in smaller increments. My husband grieves his daughter's brief life and death, but he isn't going to write a poem or make a painting to process that grief. Men and women are different, and we walked through our initial mourning alone, handling each moment the best way that we could. As my grief mellowed a bit, and he processed some of his grief, we have caught up as a couple.

He and I did not talk much about the miscarriages. I don't think that men can understand the physical grief and physical hormonal response to these pregnancies. I do think that they grieve, but in a different way. I reach out to my friends and therapist.

It has been difficult to support my toddler through his own grief. Mary Rose was a big part of his life, even for those few hours she was with us in the house. Explaining death to a young child is so hard. My son was very close to me in the aftermath of his sister's death and I let him stay close until he recovered a bit from the trauma and stress of the pregnancy and meeting Mary Rose and letting her go. I did what I had to do for my son, but I think that others thought that I was babying my toddler who faced death so young. He has a different perspective of life. For example, he says "Mommy, I want to die. I want to be with my sister, Mary Rose." I understand what he is saying, but someone else might be alarmed by his statements. I don't treat death as a bad thing, so he knows that it is part of life and that we will die when it is our time.

Pregnancy and infant losses affect a family significantly. If people are kind and continue to process and discuss things together, I think that in most cases they come back together at some point. It takes some patience. It takes understanding of our living children and our partners. It takes a lot of love.

*

LINDA BATEMAN GOMEZ
Linda's 8-week-old son Chad
died in 1986 from SIDS

Actually, I would say every family member, friend and especially my children. And I mean this in a positive way. I feel like after the loss of a child, as a parent you feel deeply that this should never happen. Your children should always outlive you. I really feel like you look at life differently. You appreciate everyone, every moment and life in general more. It is easier to put things into perspective after the loss of a child and really value every second with people you love. So for me, I feel like relationships were impacted but for the better, I don't take anyone for granted, especially my children.

*

MARY LEE CLAFLIN
Mary Lee's 2-month-old grandson Lane
died in 1998 from carbon monoxide poisoning

Probably my son. He and I deal with grief differently. I get sad, depressed, cry and want to talk. My son on the other hand hides his grief internally. He does not want to talk about Lane. He did not want anyone to talk about him. For years, Lane's name was not mentioned in front of Rob. I believe the hurt was so great for him that he was not able to talk about the baby. He loved this child so much and I think he felt he needed to be strong for the rest of us. To this day, eighteen years later, we still don't discuss Lane.

*

ANNAH ELIZABETH
Annah Elizabeth's son Gavin Michael aspirated on his meconium
during delivery in 1990 and died 26 minutes following his birth

I do not have any relationships that have been negatively impacted as result of my son's death. That said, there are certainly associations that I've had to put into perspective.

121

Shortly after Gavin's obituary appeared in our local paper, I received a pamphlet from a religious organization that claimed my child had been sacrificed for my sins. I initially felt a stabbing pain and an overwhelming sense of guilt. I quickly realized that I didn't believe that logic one bit and I tossed that brochure into the trash. I still feel a little bit of anger toward this group's practice because I believe it to be controlling (fear is a great motivator to keep us close) and hurtful. I could have chosen to stereotype all members of this faith as cruel and unreasonable, yet I chose to discard this sect's opinion, respect its members' rights to their own judgments, and then to accept that I do not have to adopt their beliefs.

I have family members who, twenty-five years following the funeral, still refuse to acknowledge my son, even when his name comes up in conversation. In the early years, this felt personal, as if my struggle and pain were being ignored. It felt like my child's life was being denied.

Whereas I could have continued the conflict by feeding into these lines of thought and emotion, I chose to recognize that everyone grieves differently and that everyone suffers in their own way. By choosing to make their choices about them instead of about me, I found it easier to avoid being hurt as result of their silence. Changing my own thoughts and fully appreciating those who can and will share my son with me has avoided the ultimate demise of those other associations. Choosing appreciation and choosing to share the joyous side of my son's life with others has allowed me to maintain those relationships in a way I can be okay with. It might be different from the connection I might have initially desired, but for me it is better than the alternative, which would mean no or conflict-riddled relationships with these individuals.

*
RENEE FORD-ROMERO
Renee's son Diego was stillborn due to
an undiagnosed cardiac fibroma in 2014

I have done so much reflecting on relationships, almost to a fault. I have been guilty of overthinking, overanalyzing what people say or don't say, the way people responded or didn't, the way people seemed to drop off the planet or how new friendships formed from heartache.

Every single relationship has changed because I am not the same. There was a distance between my husband and me after we lost our son; we're still struggling to overcome this. My husband is the kindest, most gentle man I've ever met. He's a wonderful father and provider, and he's been my partner and best friend for nineteen years. This man would never, ever hurt me on purpose. But the pressure to conceive, to replace was what was lost, created a cycle of rejection and anger that was so damaging to us both. This summer we attended a marriage retreat where some very wise mentors were teaching on how God's design for marriage is laid out in Genesis in the Garden of Eden. We studied together and the Lord revealed to both of us how we had greatly hurt each other. My husband purposely rejected me during ovulation because he was still grieving and afraid of another loss. I would deny him sex because of my being hurt, only showing him affection during ovulation because I was absolutely obsessed with becoming pregnant again. The cycle went on for a year, but at that retreat it was so obvious. We're so grateful that because we were obedient toward nurturing our relationship, even through this fiery trial, God opened our eyes and put us on a path to heal together.

God is not only restoring my marriage, but He continues to heal me through new relationships with amazing women. Women who have had similar hurts, but always seem to know the right thing to say. I get calls, text messages, and emails regularly from women who have had similar experiences, and it's always at exactly the right time. I've received two very sweet cards from the same woman, both in God's perfect time. The first was a sympathy card with Scriptures and a reminder that she was praying for me, that she understood my pain, and that she was there for me if I needed anything. The second one was really special; a defining moment for me in my spiritual walk, and understanding my purpose. Although this woman didn't know I had lost twins that time, God put on her heart to share that she had lost twins who would have just turned twenty-nine years old. God used her to help heal me, and to confirm that He connects us on purpose.

My sister-in-law recently referred to the church as "ground zero" for loss during a conversation we were having about God's divine connections with our Christian sisters. It got me thinking and praying again about how common this is, and about how lasting the effects can be. I like statistics so I started researching a bit, and I found that one in four women will experience a pregnancy loss or stillbirth in their lifetime. I would guess that just like my friend, each of those women would know how old that child would be today. According to the March of Dimes, one in one hundred and sixty births are stillbirths (that's after twenty weeks gestation). Just over four million babies are born every year in the United States, that's twenty-five thousand families a year that will leave the hospital empty handed. I know what that feels like, and I know how God used His daughters to help ME get through it. I wonder what kind of support system these other mommies have. I know the kind I have: spiritual mothers and sisters who prayed, fed, cleaned, and did anything else I needed when it felt impossible to breathe.

Do these other mommies know there's a Father in Heaven who loves them? Do they know they will be reunited with their children one day? My relationship with my Heavenly Father, my Daddy God, has changed more than any friend or relative but only because I've never been on my knees this much. I realize He hasn't changed, but I have. And He gives me the strength and courage to help strengthen and encourage my sisters.

*

BELINDA LUNA
Belinda's full-term baby Elijah
died in utero in 2012 from trisomy 18

It has impacted my relationship with my living children because I now have a huge fear that something might happen to them. So I tend to be too overprotective at times, causing some frustration and conflict with them. I'm afraid in general that I will lose those closest to me. I think it's just coming from a very vulnerable place where I ultimately realize how little control I really have.

*

MELISSA MEAD
Melissa's 13-month-old son
William died in 2014 from sepsis

Since losing William I have felt a huge disconnect with not just those closest to me but everyone. I feel as though I am in my own little bubble. No one can understand my pain because it is mine alone. I also understand that the pain William's father feels is his pain and I cannot possibly fathom how that impacts him mentally, only what he allows himself to display.

Therefore, the person that I have found losing William has affected my relationship with is his father. Although it would take an atomic bomb to separate us, we have an unrelenting bond that will only strengthen as time passes. He is, after all, half of my memories of William. To lose him would be like losing a part of William.

That said, we grieve in very different ways. I struggle to curtail my emotions most days, and he struggles desperately to cope with me, especially when my thoughts are at their darkest. He of course understands, because we are grieving the same person. But it is very hard, in fact impossible to support another person when you can barely support yourself. All you can do is physically be "there."

*

SUSAN WILLIAMS
Susan's 2-month-old son
Tony died in 1987 from SIDS

Stu and I were connected until after the funeral of Tony. Within two weeks, both of us were back at work and a sitter was found for Zach. Family and friends thought we would get back to normal, but we were anything BUT normal. During our workday, both of us put on our "normal mask" so our colleagues and managers wouldn't think we needed any time off. We were worried about finances. We had so much stress already, losing a job would have destroyed what little we had. As it turned out, three months later we were robbed of everything we owned. As devastating as that was, it taught me to never get attached to anything again. I can honestly say that if something gets broken or lost I initially will be sad, but it does not cause me sorrow or anger. My priorities had changed drastically within three months.

Work consumed me. It bled every ounce of energy I had. After work, I immediately picked up Zach from the sitter. When we arrived home, my mask would come off. I just wanted to lie down and sleep until the next day. Zach would not let me. I needed to feed him, play with him, and put him to bed with a story. He kept me alive. I had only one purpose in life at that time: to be a good mom to Zach. I can't say that I always was. I remember struggling to get macaroni and cheese on his highchair for him to eat. I also remember getting angry at him just because I was exhausted. I am grateful he was too young to remember these moments in his life.

I am not proud of myself for disconnecting from Stu, but I figured he would understand. The problem was, he also needed compassion and love. I just couldn't give it to him. I had nothing left to give. I wasn't able to care for myself. I was constantly sick and going on numerous antibiotics. We had trouble paying the doctor because of our other bills and funeral costs.

As time went on, Stu and I had some good times, but a majority of the time was a downward spiral for me. Eventually, we would turn to counseling. It helped for a time, but we needed another round about four years after that initial round.

In my opinion, even in the best marriages, the death of a child will bring both parents to their knees. Both parents have to love the other enough to know when they are having a grief moment, day, year. This is so difficult because you want to make it better for your spouse. The journey Stu and I continue to be on has gotten so much easier. My love for him overcame the moments I wanted to give up, and there were many. Zach deserved to live with both of us, and he needed us to do the best we could to be a family. None of us wanted a family without Tony, but we didn't have a choice.

After the anger of coming to grips with that reality, we embraced a new normal. Shortly after that, we connected enough to think about having another child. For me, it was two years.

*

Are there Valentines in Heaven?
Are there Red Hearts everywhere?
Do they line the Golden Streets,
Or is that very rare?
I wish that I could send you one,
Right through Heaven's Gate,
To say how much we miss you,
On this special date.
I'd like to send a Candy Heart,
That is printed, "I Luv U",
And maybe you would whisper back,
"I know, I Luv U too."
MARILYN ROLLINS

*

CHAPTER TWELVE

THE FAITH

Love is the only law capable of transforming grief into hope. -LYNDA CHELDELIN FELL

Grief has far-reaching effects in most areas of our life, including faith. For some, our faith can deepen as it becomes a safe haven for our sorrow. For others, it can be a source of disappointment, leading to fractured beliefs. One commonality among the bereaved is that faith is often altered one way or the other. Has your loss affected your faith or beliefs?

*

DIANNA VAGIANOS ARMENTROUT
Dianna lost her newborn baby
Mary Rose in 2014 to trisomy 18

What is left after a pregnancy ends without the child? What is left when a newborn dies? I am thinking of Jean Valentine's poem "I Came to You" when she says, "Lord come. We were sad on the ground. Lord Come." The losses that I write about have knocked me to the ground. My babies are in the ground. I have been on the ground, hands in the dirt, sifting through muck, planting a seed, feeding a plant. My faith is intact. Parents have been burying their children since the beginning of our history. I accept my path and my soul contract with Mary Rose. We have work to do together joined in love. We could not do this work if she had lived.

My faith is strong and will not waiver because I believe that life and death are inextricably linked together. I am not Creator who sees all. Do I understand why my womb has been emptied without a healthy breathing child three times? I can only understand a fragment. I do not understand why there is so much loss in our lives, but I believe in karma and the afterlife, and I know that this earth plane is not all that there is. To carry a child like Mary Rose, is to carry light. She heals others now. She is with us.

All of this grief, all this loss of the family I imagined, the pregnancies I desired, the daughter I always wanted to raise has given me a new attitude. I don't fuss about things that used to matter, like a broken dish or sticks in my yard. I have been put into a centrifuge, and my losses have spun me. My molecules are altered. My ego is being chaffed away as I accept my life as it is. I accept Mary Rose and her fragile, short life. I accept the miscarriages. I accept my living son. I am blessed and loved.

*

LINDA BATEMAN GOMEZ
Linda's 8-week-old son Chad
died in 1986 from SIDS

My faith is stronger now than ever before. However, it doesn't mean I didn't feel angry at God at times. I would pray and cry and ask him why. I would be angry and then pray to God to forgive me for questioning him, and then cry. I was so confused because it didn't make sense that God would take a child that was so loved and let other children suffer in horrible conditions? I had a million questions and no answers. I wanted answers and, of course, only God knows the plan.

It was also hard when well-meaning friends and family would try to comfort me by saying all the things I had always believed like, "God has a plan." Or, one of my favorites, "Chad is in a better place now." Frankly, that one always bothered me and yet I knew and understood what they meant. But I didn't care if it was a better place. Perhaps it was selfish but the mother in me wanted him, I wasn't ready to share him with God yet, so I struggled with that for a while. Now, my faith is stronger than ever. I know that Chad is fine and I fully expect to see him again one day. And yes, I believe in angels.

*

MARY LEE CLAFLIN
Mary Lee's 2-month-old grandson Lane
died in 1998 from carbon monoxide poisoning

My faith has never been stronger. I never once asked why. I know that bad things happen even to the best of us. Life has a way of changing right before our eyes. I don't really know how people with no faith make it through tough times, especially death. When we first got the news that there was no life left in Lane, I used my faith in God to bring me through this ordeal. I have always counted on Him during hard times and good times. It was never a one-way street. I realize that when a death occurs we all want to blame someone, even God. My faith told me that while I was crying for the loss of my grandson, God was crying as well for the loss of one of *His* children and for me as He saw me hurting.

*

ANNAH ELIZABETH
Annah Elizabeth's son Gavin Michael aspirated on his meconium
during delivery in 1990 and died 26 minutes following his birth

I no longer believe that God sits in heaven dictating what fortunes and misfortunes he will bestow upon each of us humans. I have always felt a sense of paradox surrounding organized religion but it wasn't until Gavin's death that I was able to articulate what I felt and thought. You see, there is this expression that "God isn't a cruel God, he's a loving God," but the very definition of the word "cruel" means to knowingly inflict pain on another. God would know how much suffering I would experience when my child died. Therein lies the contradiction.

Believe it or not, I didn't hit that proverbial rock bottom until almost seven years following Gavin's death; that climax came on the morning I discovered that my husband and one of my best friends were having an affair. Hours after sitting slumped against my washing machine, I knew that I had to get up and do something, ANYTHING, so I made a phone call, one that would led me to one of the greatest gifts I received on my journey to healing.

I was directed to a woman I didn't know. This theologian, whose body was riddled with something like MS, sat quietly across the room from me as I begged to understand why a loving God would continue to heap so much sh** onto one person's life. "God doesn't give us more than we can handle seems like some sick joke," I said to her, "and the joke is on me."

Her response is forever burned into my brain: "God is always with us...divine intervention is rare. He was in the room with you when you encountered abuse; He was crying out in pain with you and screaming for it to stop..." I felt giant, invisible arms wrap me in a compassionate hug and I knew...

God is a loving God. As I wrote about that passage in my memoir, I had another epiphany: Just as my loving God screams out when there is injustice or tragedy, so, too, does he jump up and down for joy in celebration when good things happen.

*

BELINDA LUNA
Belinda's full-term baby Elijah
died in utero in 2012 from trisomy 18

I don't actively practice any religion. I do believe in a higher power however, and I have had very angry moments asking why would this happen to me, to my family.

*

MELISSA MEAD
Melissa's 13-month-old son
William died in 2014 from sepsis

I am a Christian, however, I have never been an active Christian, attending church or such. I have always however, felt that I have faith, that there is something. What? I don't know, again I am open to that.

Since losing William I was often asked the question, "Has this caused you to wrestle with the thoughts about God's existence," and in all honesty it doesn't. God didn't take William. Science and doctor negligence took William. God didn't choose William. William felt poorly and those who are supposed to heal him, didn't do their jobs appropriately. Do I believe William is in heaven? Absolutely. I would hate to think that he is "nowhere." To imagine my beautiful little boy enjoying eternal happiness in a place of peace is comforting, although I will never believe that he is in a better place. The best place for William would be with his mummy. He is in a good place, but not the best place.

I wish sometimes that I had a strong belief. I see how much comfort faith gives others, how they can ask for strength and be given it. I guess a part of me is not willing to accept this help, because in doing so, it is almost allowing myself to believe or accept that William is gone. And, at the moment, I am not ready to do so. Maybe in the future, but I suspect the day I meet God is the day I meet William again.

*

SUSAN WILLIAMS
Susan's 2-month-old son
Tony died in 1987 from SIDS

I hated God. How could He do this to me? I had a student in my high school choir who was pregnant, and I went back to school in two weeks only to see her every day. I hated God. Why did He think I was such a bad mother?

This is what a cradle-Catholic in my generation believes. My faith at the time was enhancing my guilt. Father Charlevois was the priest who initially stayed with me at the hospital until Stu and my parents arrived. Waiting such a time with me had to have been so difficult for him. He continued to help me with my faith. He did not lecture me about verses in the Bible, but he did listen to me. He would ask me questions about me. He did not judge me for any of my feelings. He was just there for me. That helped a great deal.

I never stopped going to Sunday Mass but many times I had to go to the car and cry. The songs were really hard to listen to, much less sing. Christmas and Easter were acts of sacrifice. I really can't tell you how I got through those Masses. In hindsight, Jesus would have understood if I had missed. My new goal was to do anything to get to heaven so I could be with my son. If that meant going to Mass, than I had to do it. I knew my son was in heaven. He was baptized two days before he died. I would need to change my life to live with him when I died. These were the thoughts that overcame me when I was a young twenty-eight-year-old woman who just lost her second son.

The Compassionate Friends helped me to think about what I was saying about faith during their meetings. It was very helpful to hear people of different religions, or no religion, give their point of view about who God was to them. When the subject came up it gave me a chance to throw out my problems with God. It was very helpful to know many of them shared some of the pains I was going through at the time. I started to think of God as a loving God instead of a God who should be feared. It amazes me that my church did not help me come to this understanding, but the people that have the greatest reason to hate God gave me this understanding.

Currently, I facilitate for The Compassionate Friends at my church. TCF is not affiliated with any religion, but my church allows TCF to hold their meetings in one of the rooms. I have been doing this for twenty years. I'm not sure anyone (minister, priest, rabbi) can administer to a bereaved parent as well as a person who has been through the same thing. I want to help those who struggle with God. Also, it's nice to have the rest of the group give their stories as well. It is important to allow a bereaved person their own faith journey. My faith journey is amazing. I own it, and I work hard at it. I am a completely different Catholic. I have screamed, cried, cussed, and bargained with God and He still listened. He answered my prayers in His time, and it was perfect.

I will continue this faith journey. I will continue to question, disagree, fight, hurt and love God. It's just what I seem to do.

*

No one can know how much I love you,
because you are the only one who knows
what my heart sounds like from the inside.
UNKNOWN

*

CHAPTER THIRTEEN

OUR HEALTH

Health is a state of complete physical, mental, and social well-being, and not merely the absence of disease or infirmity. -WORLD HEALTH ORGANIZATION

As our anatomical and physiological systems work in tandem with our emotional well-being, when one part of our body is stressed, other parts become compromised. For some, grief leads to a total disregard of all health habits while others embrace improved health habits to help strengthen coping abilities. Has your grief affected your physical health?

*

DIANNA VAGIANOS ARMENTROUT
Dianna lost her newborn baby
Mary Rose in 2014 to trisomy 18

My body will never be the same. One strange thing that happened during my pregnancy is extreme light sensitivity which I never had before. In researching trisomy 18 for my book I found out that trisomy 18 often causes photophobia, an extreme sensitivity to light. I developed one of Mary Rose's potential symptoms. Though I am much improved, I am still recovering from the extreme back/hip/sciatic pain. I also think that my breasts will always mourn the chance to nourish their baby with sweet mother's milk. It is also taking time to lose the pregnancy weight. Sometimes I still feel postpartum, but I am working hard to recover my strength and I am getting there.

*

LINDA BATEMAN GOMEZ
Linda's 8-week-old son
died in 1986 from SIDS

After Chad died I had no interest in food and I couldn't sleep. I lost a lot of weight and I know my family was worried about me. On Sundays, the day he died, I choose not to eat at all. I'm not even sure why I did that. A protest of some sort, my own way of saying I couldn't control what happened on the horrible Sunday but I have control over what I eat? In looking back I'm not sure what the reasoning was, or if there was any. I think about those days. It is still so vivid at times that it is surprising the detail that I remember, but my actions I can't describe. I was physically and mentally drained and certainly the lack of sleep and food didn't help that situation but that too has passed. My health at age sixty is as good as it has ever been and I don't pass up meals or sleep.

*

BELINDA LUNA
Belinda's full-term baby Elijah
died in utero in 2012 from trisomy 18

Yes. I have experienced weight loss, change in appetite, anxiety and depression.

*

MELISSA MEAD
Melissa's 13-month-old son
William died in 2014 from sepsis

Yes, dramatically. Physically I went through, and am still going through, all the changes one might expect. I immediately lost a large amount of weight, with shock, not eating, stress and anxiety.

Medication forced me to eat, medication I knew I had to have or I would be hospitalized for my own safety. Prior to losing William, I had three ovarian tumors amongst other things. This left me with less than half of only one ovary. William was a miracle, literally.

William was a blessing. If I were to ever put faith in God it would be in that moment, the moment he gave me William, the moment I became his mummy. The shock and stress of losing William has forced me to go through an early menopause (so they currently think at the time of writing).

I have suffered mostly with my mental health. At times I've had uncontrollable anxiety, I could not eat, would have sever tremors, and pick my skin continuously. I have horrendous flashbacks to that moment, the moment I found him. The CPR, the call handler's voice talking through the CPR, and 1 and 2 and 3 and 4 and 1 and 2 and 3 and 4, rescue breath 1.....rescue breath 2.... and 1 and 2 and 3 and 4. All three minutes and forty four seconds of it. I can remember the digits turning over on the phone, and with every second my life slipped away.

I have completely abandoned my own health, I have no desire to look after myself. I shower and work, but I am not in a position to want to go swimming, to cook a healthy meal. To eat is a struggle. I don't think until the shock, the stress and the anxiety subsides I will be able to really tell the impact losing William has had on my physical health. All I do know is that my battle with mental health is just that, my biggest battle.

*

SUSAN WILLIAMS
Susan's 2-month-old son
Tony died in 1987 from SIDS

I was a physical mess. I ended up with many sinus infections. When you cry like I do, I'm surprised they didn't just insert a stint to hook up a hose to my nose. Because of the cost of doctor visits, prescriptions, and missing days of work I also developed an upper

GI hernia. Once that subsided, I felt a lot better. I was able to eat better, sleep better, and my depression started to taper off slowly. I have always liked to run. I like to run when I only have an hour, but I need to clear my mind. I use running to lose weight, calm my hyperactive personality, and release stress. After my physical problems got better, I turned to running again. It was just the medication I needed. All I had to say to Stu was: I need to go for a run. He was more than happy to get me out of house knowing I would come back better than when I left.

Now that I'm in my fifties, I don't run as much. I continue to do short runs, long hikes, and I have recently taken up golfing. Anything outside is helpful to me. I find myself connecting with God and I also have talks with Tony. Nature lends itself to seeing things that are meant only for you.

*

CHAPTER FOURTEEN

THE QUIET

Heavy hearts, like heavy clouds in the sky, are best
relieved by the letting go of a little water.
- ANTOINE RIVAROL

The endless void left in our precious baby's absence remains day
and night. When our minds are free from distractions there is a
moment when sorrow fills the void, threatening to overtake us,
unleashing the torrent of tears. For some, that moment happens
during the day, for others it comes at night. What time is hardest
for you?

*

DIANNA VAGIANOS ARMENTROUT
Dianna lost her newborn baby
Mary Rose in 2014 to trisomy 18

Nighttime is hardest as everyone is asleep and I can feel my
grief fully. It's not quite so bad these days, but in the postpartum
period when I was so exhausted and couldn't sleep, the nights were
challenging. I became depressed. This was also true during the
pregnancy when I faced the long nights and wondered when Mary
Rose would die and how many days I would have with her.

*

LINDA BATEMAN GOMEZ
Linda's 8-week-old son Chad
died in 1986 from SIDS

Morning, without question, it was always the morning that was the hardest time of day for me. It seemed like upon waking up, the first thing that would come to my mind was that this had really happened. It was not a nightmare, although it felt like one. It was reality, a horrible, horrible reality that my son Chad had died. It was as though the news was fresh every day, especially in the first few weeks, and it was so painful. I dreaded waking up. And then, like all things, with the passing of time, it became less and less difficult when the morning sun came through my window. As the mornings turned into sunsets, and the days into weeks, time softened the pain as only time can do. Now I look forward to mornings and all the wonders the new day brings. It does get better, it really does. Your days and your nights will be good again, it just takes the gift of time.

*

KARI BROWN
Kari's 2-year-old daughter Dominique (Deedee)
died in 2014 from obstructive sleep apnea

Immediately after the loss of our daughter, the nighttime was usually the difficult time. Dominique slept with us every night due to her medical needs. That very first night, we could not sleep because we felt so empty without her sprawled across the middle of the bed. For the first couple of months I had nightmares of her dying in our arms, and often woke up screaming "No!" The pain of her absence has eased up a little. We keep her toy in the middle of our bed still. If I am really missing her, we wrap her urn in her blanket and put it in the middle. My day-to-day life has forever changed. It was hard going from staying home to working full-time and attending school. But filling my days with work and school has only strengthened my determination to become a Registered Nurse and help others like Dominique.

*

MARY LEE CLAFLIN
Mary Lee's 2-month-old grandson Lane
died in 1998 from carbon monoxide poisoning

Nights were the hardest for me. Charmayne would take care of Lane during the day and by night she was exhausted. I would go over to their house after work each day and help with baby duty. If Lane had not been bathed which he usually was, I could give him his bath. Since Charmayne did not nurse, I got to feed him his bottle and hold him, love him, rock him. So when Lane never came home again, I had no need to go over to their house each day. The nights were long and lonely. I missed him. As much as I did not want to be a grandmother the first time, I could not wait for another grandson. Not to replace Lane but to help with the hurt and loss and bring some joy back into our lives.

*

ANNAH ELIZABETH
Annah Elizabeth's son Gavin Michael aspirated on his meconium
during delivery in 1990 and died 26 minutes following his birth

Twenty-five years have passed since Gavin's death and though there are some things that I can recall as if they happened twenty-five minutes or twenty-five days ago, there are other things that I can't resurrect. This is one of the latter. The first thought that came to mind when I read the question was, "all of them." Every. Minute. Of. Every. Day. But I honestly don't believe that to be true. If I am to step back from the emotion and look at that timeframe objectively, the hardest part of the day depended on any number of random things. The constant ache in my swollen breasts was a stark reminder that my son was gone. How much sleep I had determined how much energy I had to get through the day and how much tolerance I had to face any reminder about the past or the future I wasn't going to have. What song happened to be playing on the radio. Seeing a stroller someone had tossed to the curb like an unwanted baby might be left in a garbage can. Who phoned me to

143

ask, "How are you doing?" In what tone of voice that person asked, "How are you doing?" Who avoided the subject of my grief or my dead son. The second I spotted blood on my underwear and Lord only recalls how many hours following the start of my menstruation. Which meant I wasn't pregnant.

The Easter after my son's death, my husband gave me one of those electric bunnies that inched forward, squeaked and wiggled its whiskers. I blubbered for hours and I do mean snot-running-down-your-chin-and-onto-your-clothes sort of crying. My husband had no idea what to do to console me because he'd bought it with good intentions and a feeling that it would bring me joy. That bunny now has a special bench on my bedroom bureau.

What I do recall however, is that the silence of my thoughts was deafening in those early days and months. There were times I desperately wanted and needed someone to show up and distract me from those torturous memories that replayed without end. And all too often the hours I spent holding on for dear life before someone arrived, or the heart-twisting pain left, were some of the most difficult.

*

NEISHA HART
Neisha's 6-month-old daughter
Brimley died in 2015 to SUID

By far, the hardest time of day for me is at night. I often find myself having a hard time falling asleep because my mind often races far too much to be calmed. Shortly after our loss, I was scared to fall asleep because I would have terrible nightmares that played the day of our daughter's death over and over. Almost a year later I still find myself having a hard time falling asleep when I am alone or have had a bad day. My mind is instantly carried to Brimley and eventually sadness and tears creep in to keep me awake. It has gotten a lot better from where it started, and I hope it still continues to get better as the days and months go on.

*

BELINDA LUNA
Belinda's full-term baby Elijah
died in utero in 2012 from trisomy 18

Honestly I can't recall that there wasn't a part of the day that wasn't hard for me. I would wake up and instantly remember that I wasn't pregnant anymore and that it all felt surreal still. I would sit and stare out the window for hours. It felt like I was waiting for someone but I didn't know who. The days were long as were the nights.

*

MELISSA MEAD
Melissa's 13-month-old son
William died in 2014 from sepsis

The hardest time of day for me is the moment I wake up and begin to relive the nightmare all over again. There are no split-second moments that you believe this not to be happening. People often say to me, aren't the night times worse? But I really don't think they are. During the night you would be sleeping, William would be sleeping, I'm not doing anything I would normally do. Of course my thoughts run away with me, I think terrible things when I lay there in the dark alone, however, I think those things during the day. PTSD doesn't discriminate, it doesn't pick what time of day you are most lonely, most vulnerable. So, any time of the day can be as equally debilitating. I don't get a choice when flashbacks force my day down a different route.

In fact I think I prefer nighttime. I don't have to pretend, I don't have to join in the conversation or go and do something I really don't want to do. At nighttime, I can lay there with no mask on. I can cry. I can be alone, be at peace with my little boy with no fear of the outside world watching.

145

I have always found daytime to be the worst. Knowing that at this point during the day we would be getting changed and having breakfast together. Knowing that on the drive home I go straight over the roundabout rather than turning right to go and collect William from nursery. The impact and change affects my day-to-day life the most. Having to learn to live without him and do things differently is significantly harder than lying in bed crying.

*

SUSAN WILLIAMS
Susan's 2-month-old son
Tony died in 1987 from SIDS

An infant wakes up their mommy because they need to nurse. I continued to wake up in the evening because my body told me Tony needed to be nursed. I would cry knowing that this wasn't a dream. He truly was dead. When I got up in the morning I didn't hear him crying to nurse. Another reminder that this is another day without him in it. This was how I went to sleep and woke up every morning until my soul understood that he truly died. It was hell.

*

CHAPTER FIFTEEN

OUR FEAR

The only thing we have to fear is fear itself.
-FRANKLIN D. ROOSEVELT

Fear can cut like a knife and immobilize us like a straitjacket. It whispers to us that our lives will never be the same, our misfortunes will manifest themselves again, and that we are helpless. How do we control our fear, so it doesn't control us?

*

DIANNA VAGIANOS ARMENTROUT
Dianna lost her newborn baby
Mary Rose in 2014 to trisomy 18

I am most afraid that my son, my husband, and anyone I love will die. I am hypervigilant with every cold my son gets, and I worry that he will die from all sorts of diseases or accidents. This is part of PTSD when you lose someone. It is normal but exhausting. How can you trust life and God when something so precious has been taken away? When something life-affirming and good and bountiful becomes death? It is such a challenge for me. I am also afraid of getting pregnant again, of being pregnant, as well as not trying one more time. I don't want to regret not being pregnant again when I am older, but the thought of pregnancy is so traumatic for me, especially after the miscarriages. My fears and my anxiety are very difficult to cope with, and are not lessening yet.

147

*

LINDA BATEMAN GOMEZ
Linda's 8-week-old son Chad
died in 1986 from SIDS

My biggest fear after losing Chad was losing my other children. Prior to his death, it never once crossed my mind that one of my children could die. It seemed to me that as long as I took good care of them and watched them carefully, they would always be happy and healthy.

After Chad died, I was so focused on watching and worrying about the health and safety of my other children that I almost made them and myself crazy. I didn't want them to be out of my sight for even a second. I watched everything I fed them, I was fearful of hot dogs, peanuts, honey, anything I could think of or had ever heard of that a child could choke on or have an allergic reaction to.

While the years have softened that worry like time does for everything, I would not be honest if I don't admit that still to this day I have far more fear than I believe to be normal. My other children are all healthy adults now and yet I'm forever fearful that something might happen to one of them. When they travel especially, I do not rest until they are safely back home.

I was always a very cautious mother, even before Chad died. I do believe, however, his death caused me an increased fear for my other children and their safety. No parent ever expects to lose their child and I think when it happens, this newfound reality can increase our sense of worry, at least this has been the case for me. The fear and the worry certainly don't change anything and of course, some of that worry is just part of being a mother I suppose. Being a mother brings with it fear, worry, joy, laughter and yes, even heartbreak, but it is worth it. Motherhood is truly the most special relationship a woman could ever have.

*

MARY LEE CLAFLIN
Mary Lee's 2-month-old grandson Lane
died in 1998 from carbon monoxide poisoning

All my life I have been afraid of everything. Would I make a good grade on that test? Would I ever have a normal life? Would I ever get married? Would that lump be cancer? Would I make enough money to survive? Would people like me if I said "no" to them? I feared just about everything. After Lane died, I still feared life and all that was around me. My husband died recently and I have been grieving. The experts tell you that something good comes out of a death. Well, I no longer fear anything. I am jealous my husband is in Heaven with my grandson, but happy as well.

*

ANNAH ELIZABETH
Annah Elizabeth's son Gavin Michael aspirated on his meconium
during delivery in 1990 and died 26 minutes following his birth

This is a layered response. I do know, without a shadow of doubt, that we cannot—CANNOT—prevent tragedy or misfortune from happening. We can do everything right and still face devastating events. Every day random things happen like planes landing on houses and killing someone who just happened to take a nap on the couch. RANDOM. When my children were toddlers, many people made references that felt like they wanted me to smother my children, not allowing them to experience things, to learn their own lessons. People who knew about Gavin's death seemed to think that by becoming overprotective I could somehow shield my children from harm. I knew better and I didn't want my children living a life of fear because their brother died from some freak thing. That said, if I dig deep into some of the emotion behind some of my decisions, it was the fear of something happening to them that drove my thoughts. Because I was so in-tune with that line of thinking, however, more often than not I was able to stop that mind chatter from taking over.

*

NEISHA HART
Neisha's 6-month-old daughter
Brimley died in 2015 to SUID

The thing that I am most afraid of is being a parent again. The thought of pregnancy doesn't scare me but the fact of being home with a newborn scares me. It's not the fact that I don't think I am a good parent, or I won't be able to support my child, I think it is my thoughts that scare me the most. I am scared that I am going to have panic attacks about my child's breathing and not being about to let my child sleep in peace. It's the thought of history repeating itself that scares me the most.

*

BELINDA LUNA
Belinda's full-term baby Elijah
died in utero in 2012 from trisomy 18

I'm afraid that everyone I love and hold close to my heart will be taken from me.

*

MELISSA MEAD
Melissa's 13-month-old son
William died in 2014 from sepsis

My biggest fear is tomorrow. I know that tomorrow will be exactly the same as today. Tomorrow will also not include William. I'm not going to wake up and things will be different. They will be the same. I fear the unknown. I fear how I will feel. I fear being happy. I fear being happy without William. I fear there will be so many more days and nights the same as today.

Initially I feared that no one would know how I felt, I feared that I was alone. I know now that I'm not, I know now that there are so many people like me around the world, putting one foot in front of the other and hoping for no more. I have given up, fearing that those around me don't know how I feel, because I know they never will. Some people try to understand but they can't. You can't explain it, I hope they never have to, but I've stopped trying to explain, I've stopped worrying that they don't know or understand.

My biggest fear is somehow leaving William behind. I fight so hard to keep him alive in everyone's thoughts. I know that he will never be out of my mind but I fear people forgetting him, forgetting how wonderful he is and how beautiful he is. I fear the day that no one mentions his name, or talks about him. I pretty much fear everything, I fear life. I fear life without William.

*

A person's a person,
no matter how small.
DR. SEUSS

*

CHAPTER SIXTEEN

OUR COMFORT

Life is made up, not of great sacrifices or duties, but of little things, in which smiles and kindness, and small obligations given habitually, are what preserve the heart and secure comfort.
-HUMPHRY DAVY

Transition sometimes feels as if we have embarked on a foreign journey with no companion, compass, or light. Rather than fill our bag with necessities, we often seek to fill it with emotional items that bring us comfort as we find our way through the eye of the storm. Whether comfort comes from sleeping with our child's blanket, or performing a consoling ritual, the source of our comfort is as unique as our journey. What items or rituals brought you the most comfort after the loss of your baby?

*

DIANNA VAGIANOS ARMENTROUT
Dianna lost her newborn baby
Mary Rose in 2014 to trisomy 18

Meditating, praying, reading, and writing all comfort me. I sometimes draw and paint or color. I need that quiet time when I feel peace and light and love. I need quiet to reinforce the reality of the real meaning of life, which tells us that death is but a transition from this life to next. Death is a part of the path for all of us, not something bad that we should avoid, but a portal into a different consciousness. I am also comforted by Mary Rose, my grandmother and aunt who have passed away. I feel them close by, and I am never alone. The spiritual connection to my babies and their light is so important and helpful. They have not been obliterated, rather they are in a different realm and very near to us.

*

LINDA BATEMAN GOMEZ
Linda's 8-week-old son Chad
died in 1986 from SIDS

Rainbows brought me comfort, then and now. Shortly after Chad died, I went into the children's bathroom to get a bath ready for my girls. When I opened the door, the room was covered in rainbows. While any scientist would say it was nothing more than the light from the window hitting the water and creating this beautiful effect, I would argue that it was more than that. To me, it was a sign. It wasn't just the bright, bold colors that were being cast on the walls and fixtures that struck me. It was the feeling of calm that I felt when I entered that room and found myself surrounded by this gorgeous burst of colors.

I had been in that room hundreds of times before and never once had anything like this ever occurred before. I didn't know what or why it happened at the time, but I knew it was special. It was interesting later that evening when my husband Ernie came home from work. He immediately noticed that I seemed to be in a better place. I told him what happened and he too felt strongly it was a sign, as he had never seen any sign of a rainbow in that bathroom before, and certainly nothing like I explained to him that I saw. After that occurrence, we both saw rainbows and quite often in the strangest places, and often during times when we needed it most. Today, when I see a rainbow anywhere, it still brings me comfort. I believe in angels and signs.

*

KARI BROWN
Kari's 2-year-old daughter Dominique (Deedee)
died in 2014 from obstructive sleep apnea

I carry some of Dominique's very small toys in my purse; that brings me some comfort. I also keep a picture of her in my car and at work, a visual reminder of the happiness that she brought into our lives. I also found writing to her on the days I miss her most helps to ease my aching heart. Though I don't get a response back, I feel somewhat better knowing I have something to remember our "conversations" by. Keeping a few of her things around our apartment has brought some comfort as well; they are a visual reminder of the things she loved.

At first I did not want to share any of Dominique's belongings with anyone. But I found it brought bittersweet comfort; another child using or playing with her belongings creates a connection of sorts between that child and Dominique, as if I was sharing Dominique's love with that child and his or her family. I share now, because I want to see more of the connections that Dominique always had with people. She would share her things even if it was her favorite toy, and I felt selfish if I did not do the same. So most of Dominique's belongings bring comfort, especially her clothing that now hangs in our closet; they still smell like her.

*

MARY LEE CLAFLIN
Mary Lee's 2-month-old grandson Lane
died in 1998 from carbon monoxide poisoning

My grandson had only been dead almost three months and my son's birthday was coming up. I had been thinking what could I give him to help with the death of his first child. I went to the jewelry store and found a money clip. There was a small indention on top of the clip and I had the jeweler put a small diamond in this area. When I gave it to my son for his birthday, I wrote a short note.

I told him that one day he would probably take his son or daughter to buy ice cream. When he reached in his pocket to pay for it, he would see the diamond and remember his firstborn son. I told him to share with his child about the loss and love he had for Lane.

*

ANNAH ELIZABETH
Annah Elizabeth's son Gavin Michael aspirated on his meconium
during delivery in 1990 and died 26 minutes following his birth

Knowing that people care, that people are compassionate even if they haven't experienced what I'm going through, is one of the biggest things that gives me comfort. For me, it's the little things that have the biggest effect: the phone call or the unexpected notecard that arrives in the mail, with messages that say, "Just thinking about you." Any gesture that says, "I remember Gavin. Gavin's life matters. I'll never forget." Probably the greatest comforts, though, were the connections and sources of inspiration I encountered. I now find solace in knowing that my story and my experiences have helped and continue to help others along the paths of their own journey to healing.

*

NEISHA HART
Neisha's 6-month-old daughter
Brimley died in 2015 to SUID

My family and friends brought me a lot of comfort following our loss because we never felt alone. There were often many people over at our home, bringing us dinner, taking us out so we weren't becoming prisoners to our own thoughts. The one person who got me through the toughest times was Brad. He was the only one who truly felt the loss of Brimley as a child, and I didn't feel so alone with my thoughts. I could say one word or just start to cry and he instantly knew what I was feeling. To this day, and I think for many years to come, Brad will be my key to calmness when I get upset over the loss of my child.

*

BELINDA LUNA
Belinda's full-term baby Elijah
died in utero in 2012 from trisomy 18

Hugging my children, and seeing them smile brought me and still brings me a world of joy and comfort.

*

MELISSA MEAD
Melissa's 13-month-old son
William died in 2014 from sepsis

Soon after William died and we received his ashes, we put them into a beautiful heart. We then had a special teddy bear made to put this heart into. I cuddle this every night. I hold him really close and know he's right there with me. William's dad has mentioned to me that he tried to take the bear off me one evening whilst I was sleeping so that he could cuddle it, but he couldn't because my grip was so tight, I wouldn't let him go. Both of us have found great comfort in knowing that William is with us and we can take him to places. We recently took him to the House of Parliament when we went to meet Jeremy Hunt to talk about sepsis. We were able to take William with us. We couldn't think about leaving him behind.

*

SUSAN WILLIAMS
Susan's 2-month-old son
Tony died in 1987 from SIDS

Zach was my comfort. I could hug him when things got rough. I started to look at life from a two-year-old's perspective which can be very simple. He loved frog hunting, ninja turtles, riding the lawn mower with daddy, and his grandparents. Even though I had lost a son, I still had a son who was living. Tony could not be replaced. The sorrow that I bore losing him could not be healed by anyone but me. Zach helped in the healing process without any instructions. He was just himself. A pure and simple two-year-old given to Stu and me by God. The Compassionate Friends also helped. Zach gave me the simple appreciation for the life I still had. The Compassionate Friends gave me the comfort that only people who have been through the same pain can give you.

Time for me to go now
I won't say goodbye
Look for me in rainbows
Way up in the sky

In the morning sunrise
When all the world is new
Just look for me and love me
As you know I loved you

Time for me to leave you
I won't say goodbye
Look for me in rainbows
High up in the sky

In the evening sunset
When all the world is through,
Just look for me and love me
And I'll be close to you

It won't be forever
The day will come and then
My loving arms will hold you
When we meet again

Time for us to part now
we won't say goodbye
Look for me in rainbows
shining in the sky.

Every waking moment
and all your whole life through
Just look for me and love me
as you know I loved you.

Just wish me to be near you,
And I'll be there with you.
CONN BERNARD

CHAPTER SEVENTEEN

OUR SILVER LINING

Even a small star shines in darkness.
-FINNISH PROVERB

In the earliest days following loss, the thought that anything good can come from our experience is beyond comprehension. Yet some say there are blessings in everything. Whether one's loss reveals the kindness of a stranger or becomes the fuel to unfurl a new leaf, each silver lining, no matter how small, yields a light in the darkness. Have you discovered a silver lining in your loss?

*

DIANNA VAGIANOS ARMENTROUT
Dianna lost her newborn baby
Mary Rose in 2014 to trisomy 18

There is a fierce, raw truth to my life. Mary Rose has given me a clarity of seeing that I didn't have before. I used to doubt myself, but after holding life and death in my arms, I am more comfortable speaking my truth. A neighbor recently told me that time heals all wounds. He was uncomfortable. He didn't know what to say after I told him that Mary Rose died after birth. I told him that this isn't really true. I will live with my grief and loss for the rest of my life. People say things to the bereaved that do not help us at all, because they are uncomfortable with death and grief. It is hard to be open and true in the space of grief, but that is what we need and crave. The honesty to say, "We don't know how you can bear this, but we are here." Sometimes sharing space is enough. Sometimes we don't need words to fill our moments after life-altering experiences.

The connections I have to others through my experiences have been soul affirming. I am blessed to know other bereaved mothers, to have a platform for my writing to speak to women in similar circumstances. My relationship with Mary Rose's midwife, Anni McLaughlin, who worked so hard for me to birth at home, is a miracle. She is a friend who witnessed one of the most sacred moments of my life. I called her with each of the two miscarriages, and she has reassured me that there could still be a healthy pregnancy. She supports my work. She is another gift that Mary Rose gave me.

Finally, my heart is more open to those with disabilities. I carried a baby with such severe disabilities that she could not breathe. How can I not be more compassionate to people with Down Syndrome or other illnesses? My life is richer now, as I open myself up to being in relationships with people I may not have paid enough attention to previously in the busyness of my life. I pay attention now. I know that life is fragile and rich and filled with life.

*

LINDA BATEMAN GOMEZ
Linda's 8-week-old son Chad
died in 1986 from SIDS

I never thought when Chad died that there was ever the possibility of a silver lining, but in fact there has been. I would say four silver linings actually, if I was counting. The first three would be the three children I had after Chad passed away. At the time Chad was born, we decided our family was complete. We had two girls and now our boy, life was perfect. We had already discussed not having any more children if the baby was a boy and, of course, he was. After Chad died I was conflicted, I felt like I needed to have another child right away, I'm not even sure why I felt so strongly but then there was guilt because I didn't want it to seem like I was trying to replace him. I wasn't of course, but the desire to have a baby was overwhelming. Perhaps I thought that would help my pain some, and in my case in some ways maybe it did.

I became pregnant and it did make me focus on being healthier, not for my sake but for the new baby. When Ashley was born, just over a year after Chad died, she was on a monitor with heart/apnea problems. I was obsessed with taking care of her, Tiffany and Krystle. Ashley was a little bundle of energy and was a positive light in the midst of what had been such a painful and terrible time for the family. The girls adored her and as with all new babies there was laughter and happiness. The grieving moments would hit at unexpected times and the fear of something happening to Ashley was stressful, but her birth and life was a silver lining and still is. She is an amazing adult and is making a positive impact on society.

My silver linings did not stop with Ashley. In the years that followed I had two boys, Austin and Hunter, again both amazing young men, kind and generous. They too have and will continue to have a positive impact on the world.

I mentioned a fourth silver lining and that was not a child but a change in myself. I always tried and thought of myself as a positive person but I know now, I am far better at seeing things in a different light.

I think having lost a child, I now view life and people in a very different way. I don't take time with people for granted. I don't think they will be around forever because we really don't know what will happen tomorrow. And I try to focus on the positives in life and realize as cliché as it is, as long as you have your health and no one dies, everything else is fixable. So, as odd as it sounds, having lost my precious baby probably made me a better person and that is another gift from him.

*

MARY LEE CLAFLIN
Mary Lee's 2-month-old grandson Lane
died in 1998 from carbon monoxide poisoning

When my grandson died at two months of age, I could not understand why. How was I to make sense of this loss? I had heard of babies dying of SIDS, but a baby dying of carbon monoxide poisoning? People had detectors in their home. This was one of those deaths that "might have," "could have," or "should have," not happened. After I stopped trying to fix it and understand why, I knew I would need to let it go in order to survive.

Like all of us, babies come here with something to teach us. When their job is finished, no matter how long or short, they leave us. Because of the hurt, sometimes it is hard to see what they taught us. Years later I realized Lane taught me to cherish people, love them unconditionally and to appreciate what life offers us. He showed me how short life can be and to take advantage of every moment. This was a healthy baby for two months, two weeks and two days. No one would believe he would be gone in such a short time. It did not happen quickly but when his brother was born a year later, I saw his life as a precious gift from God.

*

ANNAH ELIZABETH
Annah Elizabeth's son Gavin Michael aspirated on his meconium
during delivery in 1990 and died 26 minutes following his birth

"Every cloud has a silver lining," is a quote as equally irritating as it is inspirational. You see, we often don't see a beneficial side effect of a difficult situation until after we've traversed that particular part of our grief journey. In the earliest days after Gavin died, and I do mean the immediate week, Warren and I wrote farewell letters to our son. Each of our letters said something along the lines that, "Your death has brought Mommy and Daddy closer together." We clung to that notion like it was some sort of lifeline, as if there *had* to be some kind of purpose in the unexpected, tragic death of our son. I mention these things because I want you, my dear journeyer, to know that it's okay if you're not in a place to see a silver lining. Shiny outlines and outcomes aren't mandatory when it comes to loss and grief.

That said, at some point along our journey we are likely to notice a sort of shift in our relationships, be it the connection with our self, our spouse, our family, our friends, or our hopes for the future, just to name a few. In my case, I knew pretty early on that I didn't want to spend a lifetime mourning my son and that I was going to figure out how to answer that one question most often asked in the face of adversity: "How am I going to survive this?"

In other words: How am I going to heal?

Were it not for Gavin's death I might never have pursued this work with The Five Facets of Healing. I have met so many beautiful people on this journey and I consider myself fortunate to have been able to affect something positive and inspirational in others' lives. My life is richer for the experiences I've stumbled into and the ones I've deliberately sought out. Sure, there is still some sorrow that shows up on a rare occasion but mostly I am grateful for the time I had with Gavin and for the many beautiful asides that have come to pass in the face of his untimely death.

One of the other side effects is that I am much more aware of life's fragility. As such, I've made it one of my mantras to try to stay in touch with life's little luxuries, those simple, fleeting moments that warm my heart or bring feelings of happiness, hope and healing.

Not that I don't still get bogged down in life's minutia from time to time — trust me when I say I still do — but I've tried to raise my awareness of life's many positive vibrations.

*

NEISHA HART
Neisha's 6-month-old daughter
Brimley died in 2015 to SUID

I think the silver lining that has resulted from my loss is seeing who really is there for us and who just wants to be in the picture. My relationship with Brad has become different. I think our relationship has become stronger because we are able to talk to one another and feel one another's pain that no one else will ever feel. We spend less time together now, but the time we spend together is quality time. Whereas before, we could spend all the time together and would get annoyed or frustrated with each other very quickly. That doesn't happen anymore.

I used to have very, very strong relationships with my parents. Now I don't. I barely talk to or see my parents anymore where I used to call my mom multiple times a day and look forward to when my dad would stop by unannounced. Now, I don't long for those interactions like I used to. I would rather be alone or with Brad instead of talking to or seeing my parents. I do miss the relationships I used to have with them, but don't feel as if they will ever be the same.

*

BELINDA LUNA
Belinda's full-term baby Elijah
died in utero in 2012 from trisomy 18

I do believe that this experience has shown me that in every hardship there is something positive that can be extracted. The hard part is finding the positive and knowing this lesson was dealt to you for a reason. My silver lining has been numerous things. I have learned to love more fiercely, I do not take anything for granted and I have built stronger relationships with my children here on earth. It doesn't get much better than that.

*

MELISSA MEAD
Melissa's 13-month-old son
William died in 2014 from sepsis

I don't think there is a silver lining after losing a child. The difference between now and before William died is that I am forced to look for happiness in other places. I have no choice but to live with what is now life.

I have met many friends, mostly other bereaved parents, and they have been a tremendous help. I don't like the term "silver lining," as I don't think it's possible to see it as such. You have to make the most of what you are left with, and this is deriving our needs in other places. My need as a mother to organize has manifested in organizing fundraising events in William's memory.

My need to love as a mother continues on, as the days give way to night. Time doesn't stop that bond, that love, that need to love so palpably grows. It is a tangible love that has no place to go. Therefore I feel I have to apply this elsewhere. Maybe I'm not there yet, maybe I haven't found my silver lining. Maybe I won't allow myself to have a silver lining, after all how can anything good come out of losing William? No matter of fundraising, no matter how much writing, how many people around the world learn about my beautiful little boy, it doesn't bring him back. You can't hug memories.

*

SUSAN WILLIAMS
Susan's 2-month-old son
Tony died in 1987 from SIDS

I never miss an opportunity to stop and admire beauty. This beauty can be found in a child, nature, music, art, and most of all, a loving act directed toward me. It took a long time to be able to see past my own sorrow. That is part of the grief process. Anger, bitterness, guilt, entitlement and self-centeredness took control over me for a year or two. I got to the point in my grief that I didn't like me anymore. Tony was made from the love of Stu and me. I needed to feel love again. So I needed to love again. I still struggle with love. I loved my son so much, and he died. Loving is a risk for anyone, but more so for a parent who has lost a child. Complete over-the-top love is what I'm striving for in this life. To achieve that type of love, I have to be patient.

Looking at nature with someone who sees it like I do gives me that love. I do not take advantage of compliments anymore. I say thank you. I appreciate them, and give gratitude for them. To be able to appreciate love is huge for me. To be able to say with complete honesty that I love my husband with my whole heart and soul is such a milestone for me. He is the father of all my sons. More than that, he has seen me through the worst I have ever been. Tony's death did not hurt our love, or the love we had for our other family members and friends. Love showed itself through these people. The most loving and compassionate family and friends stuck with us. I can promise you that they did not have an easy journey with us. That's what makes them such a blessing to me.

Stu and I stuck it out together as well. The journey was long, confusing and depressing. Somehow we got a ton of blessings throughout the sorrow. As time went on, the blessings were easier to see. It's almost as if Tony says to me, "Hey mom! Look at that." I have been given signs that I could not have seen early in my grief. I often heard others in my support group say that they had seen signs. I was so jealous of them. It made my bitterness worse. Over time, I have learned that love gave me the peace I needed to see the signs that Tony continues to leave me. I have also been given the gift of patience with children and geriatric adults. I can see my son in them, even if they are miserably crabby. I just sit down and ask them some questions about them. Who doesn't like to talk about themselves? I know they feel my peace when I leave them with a hug or a kiss.

I lost my son Tony twenty-eight years ago. Peace in my heart did not happen without being patient with my feelings. I needed help from others, including counselors, doctors, family and friends. I would encourage all parents, grandparents, and siblings who are stuck in raw grief for more than three years to get extra help from a counselor.

You deserve to see a light. I have a light that shines in my soul. I never thought I would ever see a light of happiness again after Tony died. My silver lining is the light that continues to shine in me. I want to share that light with others who are going through the sorrow of losing a child, grandchild or sibling. I want to let them see that their child, grandchild, or sibling can help them to get through their sorrow, and lead them toward the light.

*

If love could have saved you,
you would have lived forever.

*

CHAPTER EIGHTEEN

OUR HOPE

We have always held to the hope, the belief, the conviction that there is a better life, a better world, beyond the horizon. -FRANKLIN D. ROOSEVELT

Hope is the optimism, the fuel that urges us to get out of bed each morning and keep moving forward. It is the promise that tomorrow will be better than today. Each breath we take and each footprint we leave is a measure of hope. So is hope possible in the aftermath of loss? If so, where do we find it?

*

DIANNA VAGIANOS ARMENTROUT
Dianna lost her newborn baby
Mary Rose in 2014 to trisomy 18

Hope is being in the present moment and feeling peace regardless of what could happen but hasn't happened, regardless of what happened in the past. It is only in the present moment that I can feel hope. Hope that I will be okay, that my family is safe, that Mary Rose is not a big sadness in my life, but a gift that I will continue to share with others.

*

LINDA BATEMAN GOMEZ
Linda's 8-week-old son Chad
died in 1986 from SIDS

Hope...such an important, life-changing word. Hope offers a future that is worth hanging on for. Alongside our faith, hope is the future we move toward when our present is painful. You will find hope as you lean on others during this dark time and gain strength with their support. Hope is knowing that many have been through a similar journey and have come out on the other side.

Hope is knowing that things will get better no matter how dark they may seem. I know that losing my child was the worst time of my life, yet I made it through. Time really does heal all wounds, and we can all make it through. It is no doubt a journey however, and the patience to get through and hold on can be tough, but you too can make it through.

The pain does ease and you will find hope in unexpected places. Focus on the positive moments and soon you will see glimpses of a future that does not include sadness. Hope is finding the positive moments and having something to hold onto, through each stage of grief.

Always keep in mind that there are many others out there to help you through this time. Do not be afraid to ask for help or guidance through the more difficult moments. Hope is a helping hand to guide you through those harder days.

Many people gave me hope when I needed it the most and I am here today, stronger than ever. My hope now is that I can help someone else in their time of need. I along with all the others in this book are proof that there is life after this darkness. With hope, the darkness will fade and happiness will once again shine through.

*

KARI BROWN
Kari's 2-year-old daughter Dominique (Deedee)
died in 2014 from obstructive sleep apnea

My definition of hope is still somewhat the same: that life will continue to get better even though the heartbreak will always be with me. I have a different perspective on faith though. My daughter's middle name is Faith. When Dominique was born two months early, we had faith that things would get better and she would become healthy. She did, and was healthier than the doctors expected her to be. We had faith that she would remain healthy, and she did until the day she passed. After, we had faith in ourselves to get through this, and to turn the pain into a bittersweet happiness. We have faith that she was a blessing; she taught us what love and life are about. We changed our perspective on life, and defined what our roles are. We are here to teach, to show that there is so much more than just living life on a day-to-day basis.

*

MARY LEE CLAFLIN
Mary Lee's 2-month-old grandson Lane
died in 1998 from carbon monoxide poisoning

The dictionary says "hope is to want something to happen or be true and think that it could happen or be true." I think hope is strength that is given to us to face anything in our lives. Without hope, we would all give up and want to die. If you let yourself hope for something, you are giving yourself a reason to look forward and not backward. Hope is right up there with faith. It says in the Bible: faith, hope and love. Even though love is the greatest, you need faith and hope to make it another day.

*

ANNAH ELIZABETH
Annah Elizabeth's son Gavin Michael aspirated on his meconium
during delivery in 1990 and died 26 minutes following his birth

Hope is like a promise that we can achieve whatever it is we want to attain. It is the sense that we can realize some form of happiness when we are sad, we can shift our sorrow to joy, we can somehow make sense out of mayhem.

It's like this little knowing in our heart and in our gut that tomorrow has the ability to be different...somehow better. Hope is the belief that we can change our circumstances, resolve conflicts, and create a brighter and more fulfilling future.

*

NEISHA HART
Neisha's 6-month-old daughter
Brimley died in 2015 to SUID

I didn't think my definition of hope has changed entirely, but at least for the past year it has. I used to see hope as making dreams and goals for the future and getting happy just thinking about achieving those goals. I had already overcome so much in my life, I never once looked at these hopes and goals with the association of failure. I never saw myself failing. Currently, I feel hope when I get the urge to get out of bed. Most mornings I don't. I have to mentally exhaust myself to get myself out of bed to do the things I need to. I think my outlook on hope will go back to the way things used to be when I get a steady job using my new Bachelor's degree and Brad gets himself established in a job. But until then, hope has for sure changed for the time being.

*

BELINDA LUNA
Belinda's full-term baby Elijah
died in utero in 2012 from trisomy 18

To me hope is something that comforts me when I'm enduring something difficult in life. Hope is that little thing that keeps me pushing forward. As long as I have hope, I will always be okay. Hope is that light at the end of a long dark tunnel. It's there and its real and it guides me every day.

*

MELISSA MEAD
Melissa's 13-month-old son
William died in 2014 from sepsis

Hope for me is the hope that one day I will wake up and it will be my last, the day that I know that I will be with my little boy once again, never to be separated again. I hope that isn't too long. I hope in the meantime I can manage moment by moment, breath by breath. I hope that I can make my son proud.

I hope that William doesn't blame me, because I carry so much guilt. It might be misplaced but, as a parent, it is inevitable.

I hope that one day I can pick him up again, hope that I can see his eyes, hope that I can smell him, hope that one day I can be his mummy again, physically. I hope that my little boy hasn't forgotten me and hope that he is at the gates waiting for me.

I hope that one day I will be relieved of the sheer pain that emanates from my heart daily. I hope that one day people will understand William isn't replaceable, I don't want another child, I want the child that I had. I hope there is more understanding and compassion in a world that can sometimes feel so harsh. I hope that one day, I will close my eyes and know that when I open them, I am with my forever child. I hang on to this. This is my only hope. I hope that day is tomorrow.

*

SUSAN WILLIAMS
Susan's 2-month-old son
Tony died in 1987 from SIDS

Hope is trusting that there is a life after my life here on earth is finished. The grief journey helped me, and continues to help me see the TRUTH. No one can help you with this. It is achieved with questioning God, talking to others who have had the same type of loss, and even being angry at God. Don't worry. He can take it.

The journey ends when you die, so be patient with yourself. God knows what you have been through. He lost a son too.

*

CHAPTER NINETEEN

OUR JOURNEY

Be soft. Do not let the world make you hard. Do not
let the pain make you hate. Do not let bitterness
steal your sweetness. -KURT VONNEGUT

Every journey through loss is as unique as one's fingerprint, for we
experience different beliefs, different desires, different needs,
different tolerances, and often we walk different roads. Though we
may not see anyone else on the path, we are never truly alone for
more walk behind, beside, and in front of us. In this chapter lies the
answers to the final question posed to the writers: What would you
like the world to know about your grief journey?

*

DIANNA VAGIANOS ARMENTROUT
Dianna lost her newborn baby
Mary Rose in 2014 to trisomy 18

I would like people to know that the grief journey has been
very lonely for me and that I am tired of the lack of support in our
communities, particularly our churches and moms' groups. I
reached out to others by inviting mothers over for playdates, but
they did not reciprocate. I realize that I am the mother who walks
into the room and reminds people that their child could die. People
avoid me. They don't make eye contact. No one wants to talk about
a dead baby, let alone a miscarriage.

Grief is part of the human condition because we will all lose someone we love eventually. I want people to understand that those who opened their hearts to my pregnancy losses and my daughter, have been blessed with the love from those souls. Those who have never said Mary Rose's name have closed their hearts to the love that she offers.

I grieve and I am okay. I am processing my path while loving all of my children. Even though grief feels as heavy and thick as molasses, there is joy. There is still beauty and love all around us even though our hearts are broken.

My path is to be vulnerable and open and filled with love and kindness even though my heart has been crushed and cracked open. My heart seems bigger after these losses, and I will continue to embrace the reality of life in this broken world where awful things happen.

The sunlight shines through the trees. A white butterfly flitters by. I pause and breathe deeply in gratitude for another day, for the love that continues to deepen with my children on the other side of the veil and my son here on earth. Tonight I went for a walk with my husband and son. An eagle flew over our heads and across the lake. I live in the many layers of life that are rich with love, grief and joy, and I am blessed.

*

LINDA BATEMAN GOMEZ
Linda's 8-week-old son Chad
died in 1986 from SIDS

The most important message that I really want to share is that it does get better. That this overwhelming pain that feels like it could physically and mentally kill you really will stop. The physical ache in your heart will heal with time. You will go on to laugh and smile and say your baby's name without breaking into tears. It does get better.

It's important to understand that we all grieve differently, and if someone you love doesn't seem to be affected the same way you are, that is okay too. There is no right or wrong and you want to do what's best for you and allow others to do the same so that other relationships aren't affected. Many times the loss of a child can affect a marriage or partnership, but if you make it through this together, you will be stronger than ever. You will also become a better person because sadly you will know more than anyone else what is really important in the world. You won't get caught up in things that aren't really important. This is not to say your everyday life and little annoyances won't still be there and the fact that they are, means you are healing but your overall view of life and people and what's important will be different.

I never thought I could live through the pain but I did and it really does get better. Life is wonderful!

*

KARI BROWN
Kari's 2-year-old daughter Dominique (Deedee)
died in 2014 from obstructive sleep apnea

The journey through grief is an especially hard experience to go through. There is never an end to the journey, and the pain will always be there. It is up to me to decide what to do with the lessons I've learned through challenges. I have learned that it eases my pain to teach others and share my experience. I am still a parent, and I have the experience of raising a child for two years and four months. I have learned not to take it personally when someone says I don't have experience, because they also don't have the experience of what I've been through. It is up to me to decide how to react with regards to my daughter's death. I ask for strength similar to Dominique's to get me through the day, and for her comfort when I am having a hard day.

I miss Dominique every single second, and I long for her to be here with me. I know she is watching over me; I see signs of her everywhere almost daily. I try not to look for her, but I do keep my mind open to the love she sprinkles throughout the day. Doing so helps me get through the hard times.

I don't pay attention to what people say about how long it should take to "get over" Dominique's death. There is no expiration on grieving or missing someone; it may take one year or thirty. I will always miss the daughter who came into our world, and left too soon. She taught me more about life and love than I could have ever imagined. I am forever grateful for the short time she was here with us, and will cherish the time we had.

Mama and Daddy love you and miss you so much. We are forever blessed to have you and we think of you every single day.

*

MARY LEE CLAFLIN
Mary Lee's 2-month-old grandson Lane
died in 1998 from carbon monoxide poisoning

My grief journey is different from everyone else, just as their journey is different from mine. I have been through many deaths, heartaches and disappointments in life. I hope there will be more attention given to grieving people. There are many types of grief.

When I was divorced after twenty-five years of marriage, I was grieving for that loss. Many people said it was normal for our society to divorce. They looked at it like a passage in life, not as one grieving. You don't just love one day, grieve one day, and move on the next day. People don't really understand until they go through the grief process. I believe the deeper the love, the deeper the grief.

I was once told that the loss of a child is the worse death one can experience. I have not lost a child, just a grandson. But I can only begin to wonder how a mother can carry a child in her womb for nine months, love that baby, bond with that baby, and finally have that baby only to lose it shortly thereafter. All you dreamed for that child and the hope you had for him or her was now gone.

How does one just turn this off and get on with life? I think you must grieve for that loss and take your time. There should be no limit as to when you should be through grieving. I believe one grieves for a lifetime. You love for a lifetime and you never forget. Just because they are no longer with us physically, we never stop loving them......faith, hope and love, but the greatest of all is love.

*

ANNAH ELIZABETH
Annah Elizabeth's son Gavin Michael aspirated on his meconium during delivery in 1990 and died 26 minutes following his birth

Which one? I ask, for you see there are many paths that bring about grief and I've traveled the terrain of many types of loss, from death to disaster, from miscarriage to mental illness, from infidelity to an inferno that destroyed our family's business and rattled our financial security. My grief journeys and my quests for comfort unearthed many grief event recovery tools, a collection of which I've assembled into a resource I call "The Five Facets of Healing."

What I'd like you to know about my journey is something everyone needs to know: We can go on to live our best personal, professional, and philanthropic lives, even in the face of adversity. The five most important things I discovered are:

Chinese philosopher, Lao Tzu, once said, "The journey of a thousand miles begins with one step." We need to begin a new conversation around the meanings of and the autonomy between loss, grief, and healing. We need to know that healing doesn't mean that what happened to us is okay; it merely means that we can somehow be okay in the face of our adversity.

In order to heal, we need to identify the type(s) of loss we are experiencing as well as the minor misfortunes that we tend to overlook. I call these "The 5 Ds." They include death, despair, disaster, disease, and dysfunction.

We have everything we need to heal. In fact, we are each born with everything we need to triumph over tragedy. Though the details look differently on each one of us, *we are all born with the same five facets.* The five facets are our academic ability to learn; our ability to feel emotion; our physical environment and the physical body we are born into; our ability to connect, to relate to others; and the spirit that resides in our very epicenter.

There are five steps to help us systematically make the transition from grief to healing. Whereas we often are not in control when faced with adversity, healing is a choice that empowers us. The 5 Steps of Healing are: Choose grief. Choose acceptance. Choose your facets. Choose healing. Choose vitality.

Platitudes, quotes and clichés like, "Time heals all wounds," and, "Everything happens for a reason," all have meaning, but each and every one of them holds different meaning for each and every one of us. Whereas one phrase might bring great comfort to you, it might elicit great angst in another. The reason for this is that we each bring to the table different experiences, different expectations, and different belief systems. We need to create our own set of power mantras, personal sound bites that feed our souls and fuel our inspiration. By establishing our own power mantras we establish inspiration that we, as an individual, can live by.

*

RENEE FORD-ROMERO
Renee's son Diego was stillborn due
to an undiagnosed cardiac fibroma in 2014

The journey is never-ending. I think of my babies daily. Although I will never understand why there's been so much loss and so much pain, I've stopped asking that question. There is no answer. There are women right now who are in the middle of circumstances so horrific that they do not believe that God could even bring them out of it, let alone use it for good. That notion is offensive to them and trust me, I get it! How could God possibly use their illness, their grief, their broken relationship, abuse, financial ruin for good?? I continue to pray that God will use me, to use my grief for His purpose to help other women. He keeps showing me the word JOY. And I'm like, really God?!?!?, says the smart-alleck in me. Joy without the happy ending? But in obedience, I looked it up in the dictionary. Merriam-Webster defines joy as "the emotion evoked by well-being, success, or good fortune or an emotion evoked by the PROSPECT of possessing what one desires." The PROSPECT! God is faithful and I will stand on his promise. We can choose to be joyful no matter what our circumstances are.

"Though the fig tree does not bud and there are no grapes on the vines, though the olive crop fails and the fields produce no food, though there are no sheep in the pen and no cattle in the stalls, yet I will rejoice in the Lord, I will be JOYful in God my Savior. The Sovereign Lord is my strength; he makes my feet like the feet of a deer, he enables me to tread on the heights." - Habakkuk 3:17-19

*

NEISHA HART
Neisha's 6-month-old daughter
Brimley died in 2015 to SUID

I want the world to know that I have changed. I am not the same person I used to be. Since our loss, it has taken a lot for me to go out and do things again. When you have a bad day, it is a BAD DAY! And you don't get to pick and choose when they come. You have to deal with them as they come. I want my friends and family to know that I am jealous of you and your children. I think it is going to be a feeling that is around for a long time but I am learning to deal with it.

I want the world to know that you may have to treat me differently than you did before. Things we used to talk and joke about in the past may be an instant trigger for me now. But with that being said, I don't want you to be afraid to be around me because you might upset me or say the wrong things. Anyone who knows me will know that if you upset me, you will hear about it. But I am in the process of learning how to deal with things as they come, and not waiting until they blow up later down the road and have things twice as worse as they were before.

*

BELINDA LUNA
Belinda's full-term baby Elijah
died in utero in 2012 from trisomy 18

This journey of grief that I have been on has been so complex. It's had its ups and downs, its twists and turns. It has shown me nothing is promised and things change in the blink of an eye. It's a pain like no other in the world and accepting it was very hard for me. It has changed me and everything about me as a person. But it has changed me for the better and made me stronger. In this journey of life there is always beauty in things that might seem ugly. But with perseverance and hope you get through day by day, one foot in front of the other.

*

MELISSA MEAD
Melissa's 13-month-old son
William died in 2014 from sepsis

Grief is pain, and it is undoubtedly a personal experience. It cannot be compared, it cannot be changed or hurried up, and most of all it cannot be fixed. I believe there to be a common trend with friends and family of the bereaved the need and desire to want to make it right somehow, or to make it better somehow. There is no advice that anyone can give to a mother who has lost her child to change the way she thinks. All that is required is compassion, love and to simply be there. Don't ask if you would like to cook me dinner, I will inevitably say no. Just do it, take the choice away from me. Don't ask if I would like some fresh air, I don't. Moving is an achievement. Instead find a reason why I need to go outside. Don't try and reason with me, you cannot reason with a person that has lost their child. I think the most painful phrase I was told was that it's selfish to commit suicide. Why? Isn't it selfish to ask me to continue to live a life of pain to save you from more suffering?

As a mother who lost her most precious baby, initially it was impossible for me to think of anyone else, or support anyone else, when I couldn't support myself. It's a common misconception that when two parents lose their child that they must support each other. You physically can't. You are both grieving the same person, and you grieve in different ways. William's father had to keep busy, had to distract himself, whereas I lost hours and days just staring out of the window.

The only thing you can do is to simply be there. Be gentle. Be patient. Be compassionate. Be proactive and reactive and remember that once the funeral has taken place, any investigations carried out, you don't get closure. I don't suddenly wake up the next day after the inquest happened and think, "Oh, I feel better today." It's simply not true.

Every birthday, every anniversary, every Christmas is going to be difficult, not just the first ones. I miss him just as much if not more every consecutive day. As every day becomes yesterday, it is just more time since I held my little boy. It becomes harder, but easier to function. The pain doesn't lessen, you just somehow manage to live with it. Don't ask me how I cope, because I don't know. Don't say to me, "Oh, I don't think I would cope." That is somehow like saying that I am managing to cope with something that I shouldn't be. I haven't just lost my son, I've lost his future, my future, our future. Grief is a life sentence.

*

SUSAN WILLIAMS
Susan's 2-month-old son
Tony died in 1987 from SIDS

No one can replace my Tony. I love all my sons. I feel robbed that I was not able to be a mommy to Tony for more than ten weeks. I am still a mom to Zach and Ben. They are adults, but I am still their mother. I feel blessed that I was able to raise them with their father in a loving home. It would not have mattered whether I had fifteen more children after Tony, I would still have the sorrow I continue to have every day. It is not as raw, or painful as it used to be, but it is there.

The sorrow can be a good thing. Crazy, huh? Yes, sorrow can be a good thing. It gives you appreciation for the things you took for granted before the death of your child. I have compassion. Compassion is a gift. You know what to say to someone who is hurting. You also know what NOT to say. I did not know those things before I lost my son. Remember that people DON'T know what to say to you when your child dies. Try not to get caught up in what people said wrong. Try to remember that they were there. It was difficult for them to be with you. They were uncomfortable. They didn't lose a child. They are afraid because now they are susceptible to knowing what it feels like (even though they really don't know....thank God).

Just love them where they are. Love yourself where you are. Love as much as you can. If you are so deep in sorrow that you are afraid, do not worry. I say prayers for you every night that you will be able to love again.

*

CHAPTER TWENTY

FINDING THE SUNRISE

One night in my own journey, I had one of *those* dreams: a vivid nightmare that stays with you. I was running westward in a frantic attempt to catch the setting sun as it descended below the horizon. Rapidly advancing from behind was nightfall; ominous and frightening. It was a pitch-black abyss. And it was coming directly for me. I ran desperately, as fast as my legs could go, toward the sunset, but my attempt was futile; it descended below the horizon, out of my reach. Oh, the looming nightfall was terrifying! But it was clear that if I wanted to ever see the sun again, I had to stop running west and instead turn around and walk east to begin my journey through the great murky abyss, the nightfall of grief. For just as there would be no rainbow without the rain, the sun rises only on the other side of night.

The message was clear: it was futile to avoid my grief. I had to allow it to swallow me whole. Then, and only then, would I find my way through it and out the other side.

I remember reading in a bereavement book that if we don't allow ourselves to experience the full scope of the journey, it will come back to bite us. I couldn't fathom how it could get any worse, but I knew I didn't want to test that theory. So I gave in and allowed my grief to swallow me whole. I allowed myself to wail on my daughter's bedroom floor. I penned my deep emotions, regardless of who might read it. I created a national radio show to openly and candidly discuss our journeys with anyone who wanted to call in. And I allowed myself to sink to the bottom of the fiery pits of hell. This, in turn, lit a fire under me, so to speak, to find a way out.

Today I'm often asked how I manage my grief so well. Some assume that because I have found peace and joy, I'm simply avoiding my grief. Others believe that because I work in the bereavement field, I'm wallowing in self-pity. Well, which is it?

Neither. I will miss my child with every breath I take. Just like you, I will always have my moments: the painful holidays, birthdays, death anniversaries, a song or smell that evokes an unexpected memory. But I have also found purpose, beauty and joy again. It takes hard work and determination to overcome profound grief, and it also takes the ability to let go and succumb to the journey. Do not be afraid of the tears, sorrow, and heartbreak; they are a natural reaction, and are imperative to your healing.

As you walk your own path, avail yourself of whatever bereavement tools might ease your discomfort, for each one was created by someone who walked in your shoes and understands the heartache. While there are many wonderful bereavement resources available, what brings comfort to one person might irritate the next. Bereavement tools are not one-size-fits-all, so if one tool doesn't work, find another.

Lastly, grief is not something we get "over," like a mountain. Rather, it is something we get "through," like the rapids of Niagara Falls. Without the kayak and paddle. And plenty of falls. But it's also survivable. And if others have survived this wretched journey, why not me? And why not you? On the following pages are the baby steps I took to put hell in my rearview mirror. They took great effort at first, and lots of patience with myself. But like any dedicated routine, it got easier over time, and the reward of finding balance in my life was worth every step.

Lynda Cheldelin Fell

1. VALIDATING OUR EMOTIONS

The first step is to validate your emotions. When we talk about our deep heartbreak, we aren't ruminating in our sorrow or feeling sorry for ourselves. By discussing it, we are actually processing it. If we aren't allowed to process it, then it becomes silent grief. Silent grief is deadly grief.

Find a friend who will patiently listen while you discuss your loss for fifteen minutes every day. Set the timer, and ask them not to say anything during those fifteen minutes. Explain that it is important for you to just ramble without interruption, guidance, or judgment. You need not have the same listener each time, but practice this step <u>every</u> day.

2. COMPASSIONATE THOUGHTS

Find yourself a quiet spot. It can be your favorite chair, in your car, in your office, or even in your garden. Then clear your head and for five minutes think nothing but compassionate thoughts about yourself. Not your spouse, not your children, not your coworkers, but yourself.

Having trouble? Fill in the blanks below, and then give yourself permission to really validate those positive qualities. Do this every day.

I have a _____

Example: good heart, gentle soul, witty personality

I make a _____

Example: good lasagna, potato salad, scrapbook, quilt

I'm a good_____

Example: friend, gardener, knitter, painter, poem writer

People would say I'm _____

Example: funny, kind, smart, gentle, generous, humble, creative

3. TENDER LOVING CARE

While grieving, it is important to consider yourself in the intensive care unit of Grief United Hospital, and treat accordingly. How would nurses treat you if you were their patient in the ICU? They would be compassionate, gentle, and allow for plenty of rest. That is exactly how you should treat yourself. Also, consider soothing your physical self with TLC as an attentive way to honor your emotional pain. This doesn't mean you have to book an expensive massage. If wearing fuzzy blue socks offers a smidgen of comfort, then wear them unabashedly. If whipped cream on your cocoa offers a morsel of pleasure, then indulge unapologetically.

Treating our five senses to anything that offers a perception of delight might not erase the emotional heartache, but it will offer a reminder that not all pleasure is lost. List five ways you can offer yourself tender loving care, and then incorporate at least three into your day, every day. With practice, the awareness of delight eventually becomes effortless, and is an important step toward regaining joy.

TLC suggestions:

- Shower or bathe with a lovely scented soap

- Soak in a warm tub with Epsom salts or a splash of bath oil

- Wear a pair of extra soft socks

- Light a fragrant candle

- Listen to relaxing music

- Apply a rich lotion to your skin before bed

- Indulge in a few bites of your favorite treat

- Enjoy a mug of your favorite soothing herbal tea

- Add whipped cream to a steaming mug of cocoa

- _____

- _____

4. SEE THE BEAUTY

Listening to the birds outside my bedroom window every morning was something I had loved since childhood. But when Aly died, I found myself deaf and blind to the beauty around me. My world had become colorless and silent. On one particular morning as I struggled to get out of bed, I halfheartedly noticed the birds chirping outside my bedroom window. My heart sank as I realized that they had been chirping all along, but I was now deaf to their morning melody. Panic set in as I concluded that I would never enjoy life's beauty ever again. Briefly entertaining suicide to escape the profound pain, I quickly ruled it out. My family had been through so much already; I couldn't dump further pain on them. But in order to survive the heartbreak, I had to find a way to allow beauty back into my life.

So on that particular morning as I lay in bed, I forced myself to listen and really *hear* the birds. Every morning from that point forward, I repeated that same exercise. With persistent practice, it became easier and then eventually effortless to appreciate the birds' chirping and singsongs. Glorious beauty and sounds have once again returned to my world.

Profound grief can appear to rob our world of all beauty. Yet the truth is, and despite our suffering, beauty continues to surround us. The birds continue to sing, flowers continue to bloom, the surf continues to ebb and flow. Reconnecting to our surroundings helps us to reintegrate back into our environment.

Begin by acknowledging one small pleasantry each day. Perhaps your ears register the sound of singing birds. Or you catch the faint scent of warm cookies as you walk past a bakery. Or notice the sun's illumination of a nearby red rosebush. Give yourself permission to notice one pleasantry, and allow it to *really* register.

Here are some suggestions:

- Listen to the birds sing (hearing)
- Observe pretty cloud formations (sight)
- Visit a nearby park and listen to the children (hearing)
- Notice the pretty colors of blooming flowers (sight)
- Light a fragrant candle (scent)
- See the beauty in the sunset (sight)
- Attend a local recital, concert, play, or comedy act (hearing)
- Wear luxury socks (touch)
- Wrap yourself in a soft scarf or sweater (touch)
- Indulge in whipped cream on your cocoa (taste)
- Enjoy a Hershey's chocolate kiss (taste)

5. PROTECT YOUR HEALTH

After our daughter's accident I soon found myself fighting an assortment of viruses including head colds, stomach flus, sore throats and more, compounding my already frazzled emotions. Studies show that profound grief throws our body into "flight or fight" syndrome for months and months, which is very hard on our physical body. Thus, it becomes critical to guard our physical health. Incorporating a few changes into our daily routine feels hard at first, but soon gets easy. Plus, a stronger physical health helps to strengthen our coping skills. Below are a few suggestions to consider adding to your daily routine to help your physical self withstand the emotional upheaval.

- Practice good sleep hygiene.

- Drink plenty of water.

- Take a short walk outside every day.

- Resist simple carbohydrates (I'm a food addict, so I know that avoiding simple carbs is worth its weight in gold).

- Keep a light calendar and guard your time carefully, don't allow others to dictate and overflow your schedule.

6. FIND AN OUTLET

For a long time in the grief journey, everything is painful. In the early days, just getting out of bed and taking a shower can be exhausting. Housecleaning, grocery shopping, and routine errands often take a backseat or disappear altogether. As painful as it is, it's very important to find an outlet that gets you out of bed each day. Finding something to distract you from the pain, occupy your mind, and soothe your senses can be tricky, but possible. Performing a repetitive action can calm your mood, and even result in a new craft or gifts to give.

Beginning a new outlet may feel exhausting at first, just remember that the first step is always the hardest. And you don't have to do it forever, just focus on it for the time being. Possible activities include:

- Learn to mold chocolate or make soap.
- Learn how to bead, knit, crochet, or quilt.
- Volunteer at a local shelter.
- Learn a new sport such as golf or kayaking.
- Create a memorial garden in a forgotten part of the yard.
- Join Pinterest or a book club.
- Doodle or draw.
- Mold clay.
- Learn to scrapbook.
- Join a book club.

Grief is hell on earth. It truly is. But when walking through hell, your only option is to keep going. Eventually the hell ends, the dark night fades to dawn, and the sun begins its ascent once again.

Just keep going and you, too, will find the sunrise.

Lynda Cheldelin Fell

Be like the birds, sing after every storm.
BETH MENDE CONNY

*

MEET THE WRITERS

There's a bright future for you at every turn,
even if you miss one.

*

*

DIANNA VAGIANOS ARMENTROUT
Dianna lost her newborn baby
Mary Rose in 2014 to trisomy 18

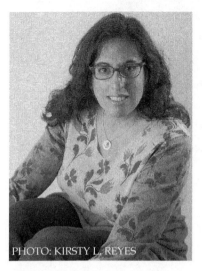

PHOTO: KIRSTY L. REYES

Dianna Vagianos Armentrout is a writer, teacher, workshop facilitator and poetry therapist.

Her book Walking the Labyrinth of My Heart: A Journey of Pregnancy, Grief and Infant Death is published by White Flowers Press.

Dianna's pregnancy with her daughter, Mary Rose, who died an hour after birth of trisomy 18, changed her life completely. Dianna wishes to change the cultural fear of death and social awkwardness around the bereaved by educating others to be present and open to the natural process of death. Not knowing what to say is fine. Let's sit together quietly not knowing what to say about our most difficult and sacred losses, because a loving community is vital to the healing of the bereaved in our broken world.

Dianna blogs about pregnancy, infant loss, grief and other topics at www.diannavagianos.com.

*
LINDA BATEMAN GOMEZ
Linda's 8-week-old son Chad died in 1986 from SIDS
Etalbeauty.com   *   Lindagomez4@yahoo.com

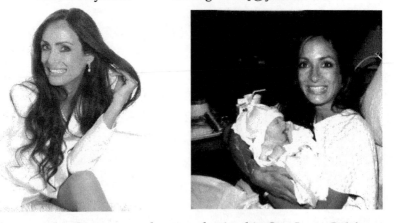

Linda Bateman Gomez was born and raised in San Jose, California. In 1975 she became a stewardess for United Airlines and married Dr. Ernesto Gomez in 1979. The mother of six (five living) very active children and two grandchildren, she is very dedicated to her children and family. In 2009, with the children grown, Linda took a step down the entrepreneurial path, becoming an inventor with a patented natural lip plumper called Fullips. As the founder of a small startup, she loves encouraging others to follow their dreams as she did and believes there is no time limit on creativity and success!

Giving back to the community is another passion. Dr. Ernesto and Linda Gomez were recognized as National Parents of the Year in 2007 by the Parents Day Council. They were also awarded the National Philanthropic Award by St. Vincent De Paul for their family food drive, raising more than 132,000 pounds of food. Additionally, Linda developed a program called Crossroads, designed to help the homeless back on their feet. This ran successfully until 1998 when the city program began. Linda is co-author of *Grief Diaries: Surviving Loss of an Infant,* and has volunteered twenty-five years for The Compassionate Friends, having lost her oldest son Chad to SIDS in 1986. Additional passions include real estate and politics.

*
KARI BROWN
Kari's 2-year-old daughter Dominique (Deedee)
died in 2014 from obstructive sleep apnea

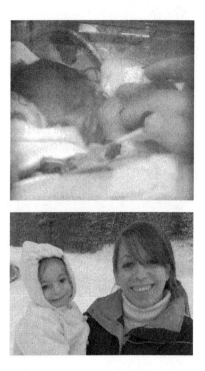
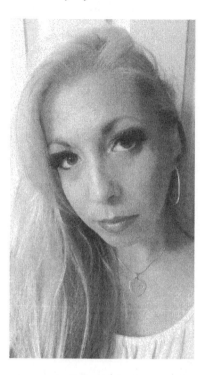

Kari Brown was born in 1988 and raised in Gray, Maine. She moved to Austin, Texas in 2008 with her fiancé Brandon.

Kari was born with Treacher Collins Syndrome, a genetic congenital disease she passed on to her daughter Dominique who was born on December 28, 2011. This was a true blessing in Kari's life and enabled her to be a stay-at-home mom while attending college to obtain her nursing degree.

*
MARY LEE CLAFLIN
Mary Lee's 2-month-old grandson Lane
died in 1998 from carbon monoxide poisoning
mlclaflin@verizon.net

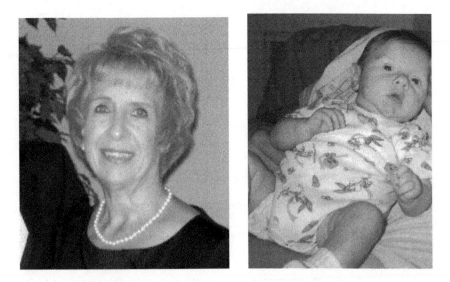

Mary Lee Claflin was born in Houston, Texas. She worked for a large Methodist Church as the business manager for over seventeen years before retiring in 2006. Mary Lee was a hospice volunteer for over seven years and sat with many people toward the end of their lives.

After having been divorced for fourteen years, Mary Lee married a friend she had known for over thirty years. They enjoyed eight wonderful years together before her husband died of cancer in 2013. She presently lives in Georgetown, Texas.

*
ANNAH ELIZABETH
Annah Elizabeth's son Gavin Michael aspirated on his meconium
during delivery in 1990 and died 26 minutes following his birth
www.TheFiveFacets.com * thefivefacets@aol.com

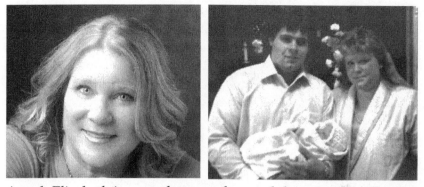

Annah Elizabeth is an author, speaker, and the creator of The Five
Facets Philosophy on Healing™, a groundbreaking guide that
helps us live our best personal, professional, and philanthropic
lives, even in the face of adversity. She authored the book, *Digging
for the Light* and is co-author of *Grief Diaries: Loss of a Child* and *Grief
Diaries: How to Help the Newly Bereaved*. Motivated by personal
tragedy, the death of her firstborn — and other big and little life
grievances including miscarriage, infidelity, and severe
depression — Annah Elizabeth set out to uncover the secrets that
allow some people to triumph over tragedy. Through her
explorations of loss, grief, and healing, Annah not only discovered
that the answers are as universal as the mystery itself, she
unearthed essential grief event recovery tools which she assembled
into an innovative program, one that teaches us how to solve grief
puzzles by identifying, evaluating, and refashioning conflicts with
intent and purpose. Annah Elizabeth's work pioneers a new
discussion and provides the roadmap that helps us make the
transition from grief to healing. Born and raised in North Carolina,
Annah currently lives in upstate New York with her husband and
numerous pets, in a soon-to-be empty nest, but that is just
geography. Annah feels at home wherever her life and work lead
her. Got Grief? Get Healing.™ with Annah Elizabeth and The Five
Facets.

*

RENEE FORD-ROMERO
Renee's son Diego was stillborn due to
an undiagnosed cardiac fibroma in 2014

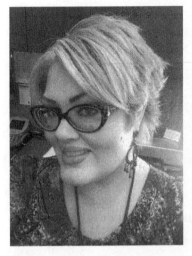

Renee Ford-Romero was raised in California's Ventura County and relocated to south Texas in 2007. She is very active in her community, serving the homeless, mentoring in a prison, planning outreach activities for her church, and participating in women's ministry. That is the work God gifted her to do, fulfilling her place in His body.

Renee is an IT Specialist for the Department of Defense, but her heart is in her volunteer work. When first asked about sharing in the Grief Diaries series, right away she knew she had to be real, honest and transparent. Renee was convinced for a very long time that she was predestined for failure and loss which lead to VERY self-destructive behavior in her teens. Trust was not easily earned because of old wounds. Pregnancy loss became almost expected but God is faithful and she stands on His promises.

*
NEISHA HART
Neisha's 6-month-old daughter
Brimley died in 2015 to SUID
www.facebook.com/brimleysmiles

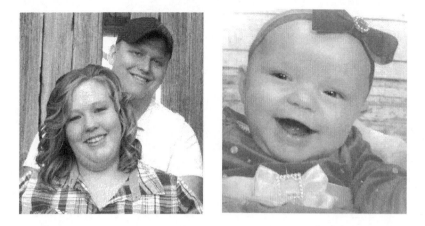

Neisha Hart considered herself an average child growing up in the small town of Marshall, Michigan. She was involved in 4-H and FFA for fifteen years. After graduating from high school, she went on to study social work at Ferris State University. During her four years at Ferris, she was a member of a social sorority, Phi Sigma Sigma, a member of the Social Work Honor Society, Phi Alpha, a member of numerous campus groups such as Social Workers Association, Active Minds, Panhellenic Council and many more.

In fall of 2012, Neisha met Brad, her best friend and other half while in Holland, Michigan, for a vacation. Once they met, they became inseparable.

*

BELINDA LUNA
Belinda's full-term baby Elijah
died in utero in 2012 from trisomy 18
belindasierra73@gmail.com

Belinda Luna was born September 25, 1973, in the small town of Hanford, California. Her family moved up north when she was ten years old and that's where she resides to this day. Belinda was married in 1994, at the age of twenty, and had two daughters during her marriage. She divorced after seven years of marriage.

In 2010, Belinda had her first son. She was surprised to find out that just a couple of years later she was going to be blessed with another baby boy. That's where her story begins and kind of ends.

*

MELISSA MEAD
Melissa's 13-month-old son William died in 2014 from sepsis
www.amotherwithoutachild.com

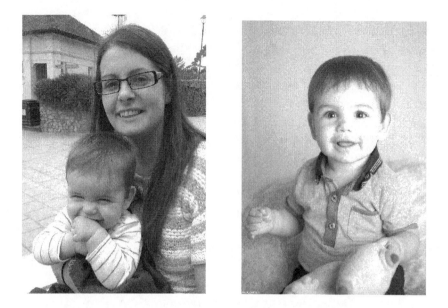

Melissa Mead was born and raised in Cornwall, England and has settled in Falmouth with her family including her partner of eleven years, Paul. She works as a personal assistant and is currently studying to become a financial adviser, she is in her last year of her economics degree.

Melissa enjoys playing the piano, although she confesses to not be very good! Melissa has found a love of writing a blog since the death of her son William as a way to organize and order her thoughts. She reaches out to many bereaved people around the world to offer comfort, and for herself to not feel so alone.

*

TAMARA NOVOTNY-KAUP
Tamara's 25-day-old daughter
Taylor Reanne died in 1995 of streptococcus

Tamara Novotny-Kaup was born in Lancaster, California, and resided in the nearby town of Palmdale until her parents divorced when she was eight years-old. Tamara lived with her mother and then her maternal grandparents until her father took custody when she was ten. Tamara's youngest brother stayed with their mother so the siblings grew up separately.

Tamara graduated high school and went on to college to study business management, switching midway to graduate from UCI with an AA degree in business communications, unable to achieve a Bachelor's degree after becoming pregnant. Tamara lost the baby and subsequently found it was difficult to find a job, an apartment and go to school full-time, so she later achieved an online certificate. A few years later, Tamara moved out to Southridge, a sub-city in Fontana, California, where she met her future husband Dave. Tamara had many odd jobs until settling in a position with the Sheriff's Department and her husband found a job in Rockwell. Soon after, they were married, bought a house in Corona where they raised the two older siblings and then had their "miracle child" Chelsey Reanne, who is now fourteen years-old and has her sister's middle name.

*

*
SUSAN WILLIAMS
Susan's 2-month-old son
Tony died in 1987 from SIDS
sueandtcf@yahoo.com

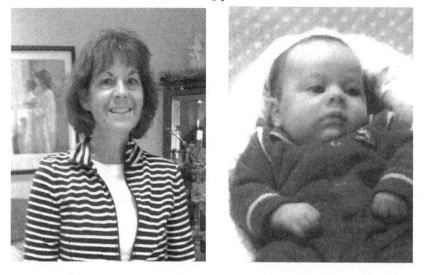

Susan Williams was the second child of six in a strict Catholic household. Her parents both graduated from Catholic colleges, and so did Susan. She graduated from the same college as her mother, and earned her degree in music education. After graduating, Susan taught music education in Indiana for thirty-three years and is now retired. One year after graduating from college, and getting a year of teaching under her belt, she married Stu. They are the parents to three sons: Zach, Tony (deceased), and Ben. Currently Zach is thirty-one and Ben is twenty-six. Both are living in their own homes in close proximity to their parents.

Stu and Sue were the first married within both families. They also had the first grandchildren. Zach was the first grandchild followed closely by Tony. When Tony died suddenly, Stu and Sue were left with the loss of their newborn son, and clinging to each other for the sake of their two-year-old, Zach. The grandparents, aunts, uncles, were also stunned by Tony's death.

One hello can change a day.
One hug can change a life.
One hope can change a destiny.
LYNDA CHELDELIN FELL

*

BY LYNDA CHELDELIN FELL

THANK YOU

I am deeply indebted to the writers who contributed to *Grief Diaries: Surviving Loss of an Infant.* It required a tremendous amount of courage to revisit such painful memories for the purpose of helping others, and the collective dedication to seeing the project to the end is a legacy to be proud of.

This book collaboration sheds crucial insight into what is often a very painful loss yet sadly remains readily dismissed by many. I'm grateful to coauthors Linda Bateman Gomez and Mary Lee Claflin for taking this leap of faith with us, and author Annah Elizabeth for helping to draft the chapter introductions. In doing so, it is our sincere hope that others who share this same path will feel less alone.

Finally, there simply are no words to express how much I love my husband Jamie, our children, and our wonderfully supportive family and friends for being there through laughter and tears, and encouraging me at every turn. None of this would have been possible without their unquestioning love that continues to surround me every day.

Lynda Cheldelin Fell

Humanity's legacy of stories and
Storytelling is the most precious we have.
All wisdom is in our stories and songs.
DORIS LESSING

*

ABOUT

LYNDA CHELDELIN FELL

Considered a pioneer in the field of inspirational hope in the aftermath of loss, Lynda Cheldelin Fell has a passion for producing ground-breaking projects that create a legacy of help, healing, and hope.

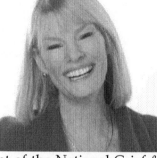

She is the creator of the anthology book series Grief Diaries, board president of the National Grief & Hope Coalition, and CEO of AlyBlue Media. She has interviewed Dr. Martin Luther King's daughter, Trayvon Martin's mother, sisters of the late Nicole Brown Simpson; Pastor Todd Burpo of Heaven is For Real, CNN commentator Dr. Ken Druck, and other societal newsmakers on finding healing and hope in the aftermath of life's harshest challenges.

Lynda's own story began in 2007, when she had an alarming dream about her young teenage daughter, Aly. In the dream, Aly was a backseat passenger in a car that veered off the road and sailed into a lake. Aly sank with the car, leaving behind an open book floating face down on the water. Two years later, Lynda's dream became reality when Aly was tragically killed as a backseat passenger in a car accident while coming home from a swim meet.

Overcome with grief, Lynda's 46-year-old husband suffered a major stroke that left him with severe disabilities, traumatically changing the family dynamics yet again.

The following year, Lynda was invited to share her remarkable story about finding hope after loss, and she accepted. That cathartic experience inspired her to create groundbreaking projects spanning national events, radio, film and books to help others who share the same journey feel less alone.

In the aftermath of losing her daughter, Lynda discovered that comforting others and sharing stories was a powerful way to help heal our own hearts. The Grief Diaries series was born and built on this belief.

Now one of the foremost grief experts in the United States, Lynda is dedicated to helping ordinary people share their own extraordinary stories of survival and hope in the aftermath of loss.

Because of that floating book her daughter left behind, Lynda now understands that the dream in 2007 was actually a glimpse into a divine plan destined to bring comfort, healing and hope to people around the world.

lynda@lyndafell.com | www.lyndafell.com | www.griefdiaries.com

GRIEF DIARIES

ABOUT THE SERIES

It's important that we share our experiences with other people. Your story will heal you, and your story will heal somebody else. -IYANLA VANZANT

Grief Diaries is a series of anthology books exploring true stories about the life's challenges and losses. Created by international bestselling author and bereaved mother Lynda Cheldelin Fell, the series began with eight titles exploring unique losses shared by people around the world while highlighting the spirit of human resiliency. Over a hundred people in six countries registered for those first eight titles, and the books were launched in December 2015. Following their release, organizations and individuals began asking Lynda to create additional titles to help raise awareness about their experiences. To date, more than 350 writers are sharing their courageous stories in thirty anthology titles now in the works.

Now a 5-star series, a portion of profits from every book in the series goes to national organizations serving those in need.

ALYBLUE MEDIA TITLES

PUBLISHED
Grief Diaries: Surviving Loss of a Spouse
Grief Diaries: Surviving Loss of a Child
Grief Diaries: Surviving Loss of a Sibling
Grief Diaries: Surviving Loss of a Parent
Grief Diaries: Surviving Loss of an Infant
Grief Diaries: Surviving Loss of a Loved One
Grief Diaries: Surviving Loss by Suicide
Grief Diaries: Surviving Loss of Health
Grief Diaries: How to Help the Newly Bereaved
Grief Diaries: Loss by Impaired Driving
Grief Diaries: Through the Eyes of an Eating Disorder
Grief Diaries: Loss by Homicide
Grief Diaries: Loss of a Pregnancy
Grief Diaries: Living with a Brain Injury
Grief Diaries: Hello from Heaven
Grammy Visits From Heaven
Faith, Grief & Pass the Chocolate Pudding

FORTHCOMING TITLES (PARTIAL LIST):
Shattered
Heaven Talks to Children
Color My Soul Whole
Grief Reiki
Grief Diaries: Through the Eyes of a Funeral Director
Grief Diaries: You're Newly Bereaved, Now What?
Grief Diaries: Life After Organ Transplant
Grief Diaries: Raising a Disabled Child
Grief Diaries: Living with Rheumatic Disease
Grief Diaries: Through the Eyes of Cancer
Grief Diaries: Loss of a Client
Grief Diaries: Poetry & Prose and More
Grief Diaries Life After Rape
Grief Diaries: Living with Mental Illness
Grief Diaries: Through the Eyes of D.I.D.
Grief Diaries: Living with PTSD
Grief Diaries: Living with a Brain Injury
Where Have All The Children Gone: A Mother's Journey Through Complicated
Grief

ALYBLUE MEDIA

HEALING TOGETHER PROGRAM

Dedicated to raising awareness and offering comfort and hope in the aftermath of painful experiences, AlyBlue Media's Healing Together Program donates a portion of profits from each title to a national organization serving those in need.

The nonprofit recipients are determined by the writers who contribute to book series.

Treasure your relationships,
not your possessions.
ANTHONY J. D'ANGELO

*

To share your story in a Grief Diaries book,
visit www.griefdiaries.com

PUBLISHED BY ALYBLUE MEDIA
Inside every human is a story worth sharing.
www.AlyBlueMedia.com